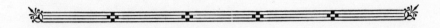

A publication in

The Langley Porter Institute
Studies in Aging

Alexander Simon, Editor

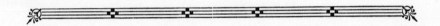

Crisis
and
Intervention

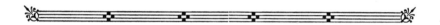

The Fate
of the
Elderly Mental Patient

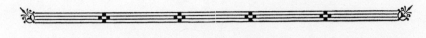

Alexander ^A Simon

Marjorie Fiske Lowenthal

Leon J. Epstein

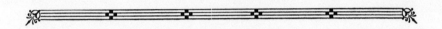

In collaboration with

Betsy Robinson

Clayton Haven

and

Gerard Brissette

CRISIS
AND
INTERVENTION

Jossey-Bass Inc., Publishers
615 Montgomery Street • San Francisco • 1970

CRISIS AND INTERVENTION
The Fate of the Elderly Mental Patient
          by Alexander Simon, Marjorie Fiske Lowenthal, Leon J. Epstein

Copyright © 1970 by Jossey-Bass, Inc., Publishers

Jossey-Bass, Inc., Publishers
615 Montgomery Street
San Francisco, California 94111

Library of Congress Catalog Card Number 75–92892

International Standard Book Number ISBN 0–87589–061–X

Manufactured in the United States of America
          Composed and printed by York Composition Company, Inc.
          Bound by Chas. H. Bohn & Co., Inc.

JACKET DESIGN BY WILLI BAUM, SAN FRANCISCO

FIRST EDITION

Code 7015

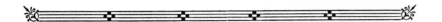

THE JOSSEY-BASS BEHAVIORAL SCIENCE SERIES

General Editors

WILLIAM E. HENRY
University of Chicago

NEVITT SANFORD
Wright Institute, Berkeley

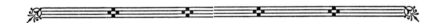

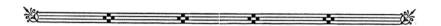

Preface

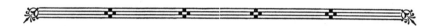

Crisis and Intervention has grown out of a series of interdisciplinary geriatric studies conducted at the Langley Porter Neuropsychiatric Institute, California Department of Mental Hygiene, and the Department of Psychiatry, University of California School of Medicine, San Francisco. The program was supported primarily by grants from the National Institute of Mental Health,[1] with supplementary funds contributed by the California Department of Mental Hygiene. Alexander Simon, Medical Director of Langley Porter Neuropsychiatric Institute and Chairman of the Department of Psychiatry, and Marjorie Fiske Lowenthal, Director of the Adult Development Program, University of California Medical Center, were co-principal investigators of the program. Previous publications based on this research are listed in Appendix E.

[1] United States Public Health Service, National Institute of Mental Health Grant MH 09145.

This book has been a collaborative enterprise. The authors express their appreciation for helpful consultations with Robert Butler, Robert Cohn, Alvin Goldfarb, Oscar Kaplan, and Walter Obrist. In this, as in other segments of the research, the intellectual and administrative support of Richard H. Williams, former Chief of the Professional Services Branch and now Special Assistant to the Director for International Activities, National Institute of Mental Health, has been invaluable. (Other consultants and the initial advisory committee that greatly aided in getting the study under way are listed in Appendix A.)

Psychiatrists, sociologists, psychologists, anthropologists, and social workers who collected data on which the bulk of this report rests were: Carroll Brodsky, Adolph Christ, Margaret Clark, Andrew Deskins, Alide Eberhard, Joel Fort, Ursula Gebhard, Patricia Gumrukcu, Lois Hurwitz, Helen Jambor, Doris Kashevaroff, Lawrence Katz, S. King, George LeBaron, Karen Many, Robert Mielke, Elaine Morgan, Miron Neal, Panthea Perry, Alvah Powers, Malcolm Roemer, David Ross, Mary Lou Schneider, Barbara Short, Audrey Thaman, Mella Trier, and Paul Wanner. Margaret Clark coordinated much of the field work for the two rounds of follow-up when the staff was augmented by Gordon Bermak, John Langton, Wayne Mercer, D. Jay Nichols, Robert Pierce, John Talley, and David Zapella. In addition, cooperative and efficient data processing services were provided by the University of California Survey Research Center (Berkeley), where Charles Y. Glock was director. During the period most of this work was done, Roderick Fredrickson was in charge of the service division and Charles Gehrke and Carol Thompson were responsible for servicing our computer needs.

Many taxing and vital data processing services were performed by members of the project staff. In this connection, special thanks are due to Clayton Haven (data processing coordinator) who organized all computer orders, served in a liaison capacity with staff at the computer facility, and supervised the presentation of data in tabular form. Karen Many served in a similar capacity in the initial phases of the project. Kay Anderson, Marion Beaver, Deetje Boler, Horace Cayton, George Craddock, Vernita Davidson,

Virginia Dunne, Frank Many, Fulton Mather, Betsy Robinson, and Eileen Schreffler served as research assistants.

Pauline Burt, supervisor of the secretarial staff, and Ruth Prael, Irma Stephenson, Sandra Hobart, Phyllis Ogino, Linda Shearin, Renee Crane, Santos Flores, Hannah Hamataka, Vira Hileman, Alice Klink, Starr Naines, and especially Phyllis Olsen, coped with the universal problems of seeing a manuscript through to its final stages with outstanding competence and cheerfulness. Geraldine O'Keefe served as project field secretary while the staff was in residence at the General Hospital. That the almost daily emergencies arising from the uncontrollable and unpredictable workloads did not erupt into major crises is due largely to her unruffled purposefulness.

The authors of this volume are particularly pleased to acknowledge the courtesy and cooperation of Gloria Bentinck, who was Chief of Psychiatric Services at the San Francisco General Hospital at the time the data were collected, and her staff. Despite the burdens created by overcrowded wards and overworked staff, they smoothed many paths and provided much background information during the year and a half the research team was in residence at the hospital.

The analysis and presentation of research findings went through two major phases. In the first phase, analytic work was undertaken by John Buehler, George Burnell, Robert Cahan, Guy Hamilton Crook, Jerome Fisher, Lawrence Katz, D. Jay Nichols, Robert Pierce, Lynn Reynolds, Joe Spaeth, John Talley, and Thomas Trier, in addition to the authors of this volume. Most of this material has been published in journal articles (see Appendix E). During both periods Mary Ann Esser and Gerard Brissette served as editors. The responsibility for synchronizing text, tables, footnotes, bibliography, and appendices for the final phase was assumed by Betsy Robinson.

Finally, to the hundreds of patients and their relatives, friends, and other collaterals we express our heartfelt appreciation for their remarkable cooperation. Though they must remain anonymous to our readers, to many members of the staff they have become unique individuals who captured our admiration during a time that was for them one of acute and often painful stress. If our work has contributed in any way to the improved care of successive generations of elderly patients, it is at least as much to their credit as to ours.

San Francisco
March 1970

ALEXANDER SIMON
MARJORIE FISKE LOWENTHAL
LEON J. EPSTEIN

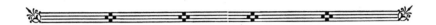

Contents

Crisis
and
Intervention

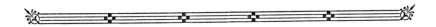

The Fate
of the
Elderly Mental Patient

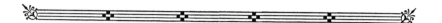

Introduction

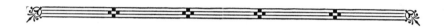

Crisis and Intervention describes a near-universe of older urban residents who were hospitalized with serious psychiatric disturbances in the course of one calendar year. Even though the psychiatric screening wards of the general hospital where they were received and the procedures used with older patients have changed considerably since the research program started—partly in consequence of this study—a description of the condition and fate over the subsequent two-year period of a number of seriously disturbed old people should serve as a useful starting point for policy planning, not only in San Francisco but also in urban areas throughout the country. Sustained efforts are now being directed, in San Francisco and other cities, toward keeping older patients out of state hospitals, but the findings presented here make it eminently clear that a high proportion of such patients benefited from hospitalization. The critical questions, which neither this study nor others have definitely answered, are whether the alternatives now available are adequate to the task of providing appropriate care for these patients, and,

1

if not, what private, community, county, and state-wide efforts will be required to make them so.

This is one of a series of four monographs and books and several articles reporting on 1,200 mentally healthy and mentally ill San Franciscans. The first monograph (Lowenthal, 1964a) focused on the social matrix within which the elderly were hospitalized for psychiatric reasons; the second (Lowenthal, Berkman, and Associates, 1967) on the mentally disturbed aged who continue to live in the community; the third (Clark and Anderson, 1967) on the personal and social systems of both well and ill. Here we describe the mental, physical, and socioeconomic conditions of one of the most deprived, impaired, and hopeless groups in our society. They were not only old, in itself not an enviable state in our culture, and mentally ill, but most of them were desperately poor, socially ignored, and seriously ill physically. During the two years in which follow-up studies were conducted, nearly half of the original sample of 534 patients died. Most members of the research staff worked in or near the psychiatric screening wards of a general hospital in a metropolitan area. Not only were the patients the most abject and destitute of all newcomers to the wards, but also the wards themselves could only degrade whatever might have been left of the human spirit: beds were so close together that there was scarcely standing room between them; there were no chairs, no place for belongings even had one not been stripped of them; there was no alternative but to sit or lie on the bed, because the wards were often so crowded that the small day rooms were also crammed with beds; the bathrooms were public and communal; commitment hearings were held at the bedside, often in the midst of commotion from other patients. We suspect that both our research priorities and our choices of procedure may, to some extent, have reflected the stresses generated by our prolonged exposure to human misery and hopelessness. Project psychiatrists who might normally have been absorbed by the analysis of individual life histories resorted to highly complex computer techniques which led them away from the individual. Some social researchers left the project to study less threatening phenomena; others, also usually fascinated by the analysis of life histories, were able to steep themselves in the project but thereafter encountered intractable writing blocks.

At the same time, becoming increasingly aware of how closely interwoven are physical and mental illness in the elderly, the staff saw a glimmer of constructive purpose in their work as plans for Medicare moved closer to reality. We could not only trace the fate of geriatric mental patients but also describe them in a manner that might contribute to plans for more adequate, comprehensive programs for their care or for preventive measures that, for some of them, might obviate the necessity for such programs. Our work might be useful for several types of readers: policy planners, at local, county, state, or national levels, concerned with prevention of incapacitating mental and physical illness and with the provision of adequate personnel and facilities; physicians, social workers, and nurses; private citizens who encounter mental disturbance among the aged with whom their own lives are intertwined. We hope also that our colleagues in social psychiatry, sociology, and psychology will find the work of substantive and methodological interest.

The broad objectives of the research program were to explore sociological, psychological, psychiatric, and physical health factors involved in the admission of older people to psychiatric facilities and to analyze, from an interdisciplinary point of view, the spectrum of normal and abnormal aging processes. Of the two original samples on which the work is based (a hospital and a community-resident sample), the 534 elderly persons admitted to the psychiatric screening wards of the San Francisco General Hospital in 1959 provide the subjects of this book. The community-resident aged whom we have studied constitute a random, stratified sample of six hundred persons drawn from the eighteen census tracts with the highest proportion of persons aged sixty and older in San Francisco. Included were census tracts with high, medium, and low rates of elderly admissions to psychiatric screening wards and with a wide range of socioeconomic status. The community sample was divided, by ratings and other measures, into the mentally well and the mentally ill. Comparisons between these two groups and the patients in the hospital sample provided a basis for studying the spectrum of normal and abnormal aging from a number of viewpoints (Lowenthal et al., 1967; Clark and Anderson, 1967). In this book, the community sample, referred to only briefly, provides a comparison group matched with the hospital sample for age, sex, and socioeconomic status, to convey a general impression of the social, physical, and functional differences between the hospitalized and those who remain in the community.

From both samples, sociological, psychological, and clinical data, both structured and open-ended, were gathered at three, approximately annual, intervals. This study design has permitted us to conduct two major types of analysis: cross-sectional (the interrelation of relevant factors as they were observed at one point in time) and longitudinal (change in relevant variables consistently observed at two annual intervals). The research program has progressed through a series of phases, each growing out of the previous one. Because of the pioneering nature of some of the work, few of the steps could have been foreseen when the original study was proposed. That this circumstance was recognized from the outset by the National Institute of Mental Health and particularly by the Professional Services Branch and its Advisory Committee and later by the California Department of Mental Hygiene, is attested by the flexibility with which they supported, both intellectually and financially, the evolving phases of the program.

Originally we planned an intensive study of a small sample of hospitalized patients. Such a sample would have been feasible, however, only if clearcut hypotheses applicable to certain diagnostic or other groups could be pinpointed as the main focal points of the study. Findings from exploratory studies conducted at the beginning of the program soon made it apparent that a broader approach was needed. The preliminary studies included analysis of admission data from the San Francisco General Hospital and from the Biostatistics Division of the California Department of Mental Hygiene of 1,700 elderly patients, exploratory interviews and examinations of seventy-five older new admissions to the screening wards, and a careful review of research in geriatric mental illness. From these explorations we concluded that elderly persons admitted to psychiatric screening wards constitute so heterogeneous a group and that so little was known about the mental illnesses of old age and their social and physical correlates that a narrow focus at the outset was unwarranted. It was clear that the original decision to study patients admitted to the screening wards rather than those admitted to state hospitals was sound, for thus we were able to identify certain prevalent types of disorder among elderly people that otherwise we might have missed: for instance, elderly persons discharged from these wards to the community were sadly neglected; some of those sent to other institutions such as general hospitals, nursing homes, and old age homes never should have arrived in the screening wards in the first place; the frequency of acute brain disorder would largely have escaped our notice.

The research staff, its advisory committee (see Appendix A), and representatives of the National Institute of Mental Health agreed at this point that what was needed most was a comprehensive body of descriptive data about a universe of elderly first admissions to a psychiatric screening ward, supplemented by information about a group of elderly persons living in the community, with and without mental impairment. Out of these descriptive studies it was expected (and these expectations have been realized) that hypotheses and research questions would develop that could then be explored more intensively with subsamples of the subjects.

Once the decision was made to embark on an extensive, descriptive study of a hospitalized sample, three major questions confronted the staff: what information, ideally, should be collected from and about the patients; how much and what kind of information could be collected with the project's budget and staff and the conditions of the psychiatric screening wards; how many subjects should be included? During a series of senior staff conferences supplemented by discussions with consultants in the various disciplines represented, it was decided that the baseline data on each patient should provide psychiatric and physical examinations and a medical history of a quality similar in detail and thoroughness to those procured at the best teaching and research institutions; a detailed report on all relevant circumstances and individuals involved in the admission of the patient to the hospital; a rudimentary life history; a health history which included both a narrative report and structured questions; a full set of socioeconomic background data; carefully selected tests of mental status and psychological condition; self-maintenance measures; a description, derived from both open-ended and structured questions, of day-to-day living patterns, including the nature and scope of social interaction and changes in activities and interests, since age fifty.

The research instruments were timed and tested in exploratory interviews with patients and collateral informants. A dress rehearsal at the hospital was scheduled for the last three months of 1958 to determine how much information could be collected, given the size of the staff and the conditions in the wards. Altogether, 173 patients were examined, tested, and interviewed in the pretest period, and an average of one collateral per patient was interviewed. As the pretest progressed, it became increasingly apparent that, with the unpredictable nature of the daily case load, either the coverage would have to be reduced or plans for studying a universe of patients would have to be modified. It became clear, also, that with only two psychiatrists, one working full-time, the other half-time, on the staff, we would have to rely on physical examinations by interns and residents on the hospital staff. Subsequently, the case load of the psychiatrists was eased by a plan that permitted Langley Porter Institute residents in psychiatry to work on the project for three months as part of their residency training in clinical psychiatric research. The two psychologists found that most patients were too disturbed by the crisis atmosphere engendered by being hospitalized to respond to personality tests and that tests of intellectual status took much longer than with normal or younger persons. Social interviewers reported that neither patients nor collaterals had the patience, at this time of tension, to cope with a detailed life history, so certain modifications were made in the interview schedule. The self-maintenance questions proved practicable and fruitful, and sociologists, psychologists, and psychiatrists spent several months elaborating and pretesting this schedule.

The decision to carry out a large-scale descriptive study does not mean that staff members were so thoroughly eclectic as to rely entirely on a fishnet approach. The medical authors hypothesized that some part of the formidable array of symptomatology often displayed by elderly persons suffering from chronic brain syndromes is psychogenic (functional or reactive) and is not a direct consequence of brain disease alone, but a reaction to it and to internal and environmental stress. This hypothesis was responsible for the use of multiple diagnoses in the research program, and has, we believe, proved fruitful. A second hypothesis was that sensory deprivation, especially a decline in or loss of eyesight or hearing, and social isolation would be strongly associated with age-linked mental disorder. A third hypothesis was that acute physical illness accompanied by symptoms of an acute brain syndrome may precipitate hospitalization and possibly affect the course of illness. The question of the relevance of other physical illness was left open but was considered a crucial area for research. A fourth hypothesis, shared by clinicians and social scientists, was that, by screening out persons who were admitted to a psychiatric facility before age sixty, we would eliminate most alcoholics and persons with other types of long-standing psychogenic disorders such as chronic schizophrenia and recurrent manic depressive illness; this hypothesis was not entirely supported by our findings. Among the hypotheses of the social scientists were: that age-linked stresses such as widowhood or retirement would be associated with the development of mental disorder in late life; that both lifelong and age-linked social isolation would be conducive to such disorders; that there would be notable sociocultural differences in the tolerance for deviant behavior in the elderly; that the presence or absence of social supports in the family or the community would have a strong bearing on disposition from the screening wards and from the state hospitals. These hypotheses were not unequivocally supported by our findings.

When a decision to aim at the originally planned sample was made, a semifinal and more streamlined battery of schedules, representing a compromise with the ideal collection, was prepared. These schedules were pretested with the next 123 elderly first admissions. After some modifications and refinements, they were put in final form, and the field work proper began on January 1, 1959 and continued throughout that year. (The research schedules we used are listed in Appendix B.)

The psychiatrists recorded their observations on a series of work sheets and included a medical history summary and reports of mental status and physical examinations. The mental status examination was based mainly on the interview and examination of the patient; the report of physical status was derived largely from interns' reports, supplemented by psychiatrists' examinations when indicated. The medical history summary was completed largely from the health schedule recorded by social interviewers on the basis of interviews with patients and their relatives or others who knew them well. On the basis of a review of these work sheets and the narrative material on the history of the illness gathered by social interviewers, the senior psychiatrist recorded psychiatric diagnoses and associated physical diagnoses, his judgment of prognosis, ratings of physical and psychological disability and activity levels, and a number of factual items about neurological signs and symptoms. Diagnoses were reviewed by a second senior psychiatrist. The few disagreements were settled in discussions with a third psychiatrist. The major innovation of this procedure for research purposes was the use of multiple diagnoses.

The psychologists administered subtests (information, comprehension, arithmetic, and digit span) of the Wechsler Adult Intelligence Scale to the 359 patients able to take such tests. Other tests administered to segments of the sample were the Kent Emergency Intelligence Scale, a Practical Functioning Scale (developed by project psychologists), a thematic apperception card that was developed for use in the University of Chicago Committee on Human Development study of aging in Kansas City, and, for a few patients, the Rorschach Test.

The social interviewers' schedules included thirty pages of prestructured questions on basic background data, major life changes, and current living conditions, which included social relationships, work history, health history, functional level. Open-ended interviews with patients and with collaterals included the following general areas: description of informant; reasons for hospitalization; participants in and consequences of present hospitalization; life prior to admission, including a description of a typical day; a brief life history; and a brief series of questions on attitudes, values, future outlook, and past and present personality and behavioral characteristics.

As a supplement to the main data-collecting operation at the San Francisco General Hospital, project psychiatrists reviewed the hospital charts after the patient's discharge. Information on treatment, laboratory findings, additional physical findings, and nurses' observations was recorded on a research schedule, primarily to provide a basis for rating change in the patient's condition during his stay in the screening wards. The project staff originally had planned to collect data relevant to change by examining and observing the patient on the last day of his stay, but marked fluctuations in admissions, with a particularly heavy influx on Mondays and after holidays, made it impossible to carry out the plan on a systematic basis. Factual data in the general schedule and in the health schedule completed by the social interviewers were recorded on the basis of "best available data." For patients who were out of contact, this usually meant reliance on information from relatives or friends or on social agency or medical records. (See Appendix C for a further discussion of this problem of inaccessible patients.) In the case of conflicting reports from patients and collaterals, every effort was made to locate a source of valid information. All schedules and narratives completed by social interviewers were reviewed in detail by the interviewer supervisor, and incomplete schedules or cases of conflicting information were returned for further checking. Relatives, friends, landlords, police officers, and social service agency and medical ward staff were, for the most part, cooperative and conscientious in their reporting. In only a few instances did interviewers sense evasiveness or discover blatant inconsistencies among the informants.

On an accessibility scale developed from replies of patients to structured and open-ended questions (Appendix C), 26 per cent were classified as accessible to all questions; 33 per cent as partially accessible; 35 per cent were inaccessible at the time of the social interview; 6 per cent could not be classified on this scale. Fortunately, only 6 per cent of the inaccessibles had no collateral informant. In most cases, collateral data were relied upon in filling out the "best available data" sections of the research schedules, while, for from one- to two-thirds of the sample, firsthand information was available about the patients' own opinions and attitudes. At least one collateral was interviewed for 89 per cent of the patients; for about one-fourth, a second informant was interviewed, and for twenty patients, three. Whenever possible, face-to-face interviews were conducted (56 per cent of all collateral interviews), but when work or family responsibilities prevented the potential informant from going to the hospital or from receiving the social interviewer in his home, telephone interviews were necessary (44 per cent). A comparison of the two types of interview indicates that, while the narrative reports of the telephone interviews were a bit shorter, there is no reason to believe that the data are any less valid than those obtained from the face-to-face interviews. More informants were available for patients in their seventies than for either younger or older people. Men were more likely than women to have no available informant. This is, no doubt, a reflection of the fact that there were more social isolates among the younger men (Lowenthal, 1964b).

For 73 per cent of all patients, relatives or, in a few instances, friends were interviewed, and for 43 per cent, the relatives included a spouse, a child, or both. Another 16 per cent had semipersonal informants (landlords, personal physicians) or impersonal ones (social service workers, managers of nursing homes, physicians in medical institutions). For 11 per cent, despite repeated efforts, no informants could be found. Of the first or "best informed" collaterals, 56 per cent had had daily contact with the patient before he was admitted; 13 per cent had had at least biweekly contact. At the other extreme, 11 per cent had seen the patient once a month or less.

When the first round of data for the hospital sample was being collected, the staff consisted of fifteen senior and junior professionals, including psychiatrists, residents in psychiatry, sociologists, social psychologists, psychologists, and social workers. From August 1958, until January 1960, most of the staff members had offices adjacent to the psychiatric wards of the San Francisco General Hospital. All members of the professional staff examined, tested, and interviewed patients.

Each weekday morning, the project secretary checked the admissions chart of the screening wards, to select a preliminary list of persons aged sixty and over to be included in the sample. Admission records were checked for eligibility criteria (a year of residence in San Francisco, no arrests or psychiatric admissions prior to age sixty, and not on a "visit" status from a state hospital). When there were any doubts about eligibility, telephone calls were made to the Biostatistical Section of the Department of Mental Hygiene for an additional check on earlier admissions. Names of persons to be included in the sample were posted on a large wall chart, and psychiatrists, psychologists, and the social interviewer coordinator were informed about the day's case load. An effort was made to examine and interview the patient as soon after his admission as possible, but because of the tremendous variation in the number of daily admissions, the actual time varied from a few hours to five or six days after admission. Similarly, the effort to have the psychiatrist, psychologist, and social interviewer all see a given patient on the same day was likely to be frustrated when case loads became especially heavy. From hospital admission, social service, and, on occasions, medical ward and social agency records, the coordinator of the social interviewers procured the names of relatives, friends, or other informed persons. If the patient was able, he told us which friends or relatives knew him best, and every effort was made to interview those well informed about the patient in general and about the events and procedures leading up to his admission on the psychiatric ward (sometimes, but by no means always, the same person). Because of the usually overcrowded and noisy screening wards, we at first tried to interview the patient either in one of our offices or in a staff or visitors' room nearer to the wards. Because patients had to be accompanied by a regular ward nurse or technician whenever they left the wards for any purpose, this procedure proved too burdensome for the already overworked screening ward staff, and most interviews with patients and most psychological tests were therefore conducted in the wards. Conditions were so crowded that the psychiatrist, social interviewer, or psychologist generally had to stand next to the patient's bed or to sit on the bed. The examiners were struck by the ability of patients, except those who were highly distractible, to cooperate with the research staff despite their surroundings. A project psychologist who compared the results of patients tested in the ward with those tested in privacy found no significant differences (Pierce, 1963).

The atmosphere throughout the first year of formal datagathering was often electric with tension. The number of eligible new patients varied from one to as many as fifteen per day. The patients themselves, and usually their relatives, were frequently in states of high tension and anxiety generated by whatever crises had brought them to the psychiatric ward and by the often devastating experience of simply being in such a ward. When the screening wards were impossibly overcrowded, the hospital staff endeavoured to discharge patients, or have them committed to state hospitals,

within one or two days of admission. This was particularly true for
alcoholics, so the research team made a point of trying to see them
as soon as possible after they were admitted for fear of a precipitous
departure. Despite weekend and evening workshifts, however, some
patients left the wards before all of the research team could interview or examine them. At the end of the data-collecting year, the
near-universe of elderly first admissions had been covered thus: 81
per cent of the 534 elderly patients comprising the sample had been
seen by the social interviewer, the psychologist and the psychiatrist;
10 per cent by the social interviewer and psychologist only; 3 per
cent by the social interviewer and psychiatrist only; 2 per cent
by the psychologist and psychiatrist only; another 2 per cent by the
social interviewer only; yet another 2 per cent by none of the research staff. No patients were seen by only the psychiatrist or only
the psychologist. Information about the nine patients in the group
who were not seen by any member of the research team came from
hospital records, social service agencies and, in one case, from collaterals. Patients for whom the coverage was only partial account
for the "unknown" category in some tables. Altogether, 96 per cent
of the patients were seen by a project social interviewer, 93 per cent
by a psychologist, and 86 per cent by a psychiatrist. In all but nine
cases, sufficient data were available from hospital records, private
physicians, and health history material gathered by the social interviewer to enable the senior project psychiatrist to assign a psychiatric diagnosis.

In addition to the varying length of stays on the screening
ward and the unpredictable daily case load, staff members had also
to cope with many requests from the hospital staff, relatives, and
friends of the patients, and the patients themselves. At first, because
of the detailed workups made by the research team, hospital staff
members were eager to discuss individual cases with the project
psychiatrists; such pressures were successfully resisted on the ground
that the research team should not influence the ordinary course of
events at the hospital any more than was absolutely necessary. Des-
perate patients and collaterals often pressed the project staff for
advice or assistance for all manner of medical, economic, and social
problems. Friends and relatives were often located for patients who
were unable to make such contact themselves; referrals were made

to the hospital social service department when necessary; crutches, hearing aids, dentures, and glasses were retrieved when possible; frequently, social interviewers explained ward and court hearing procedures to patients and relatives who were utterly bewildered by the turmoil around them. Such problems should have been handled by members of the hospital's regular professional staff, but as frequently happens the screening wards were grossly understaffed. In subsequent years this situation was, to some extent, rectified by the addition of more social workers, psychiatric residents, and interns; later still, it was markedly improved by the addition of new wards and a change of emphasis from screening to treatment. We have been fortunate enough to witness concrete ameliorative changes as the result of the findings of this research project. Since 1963, a Geriatric Screening Unit has been operating, in association with San Francisco General Hospital, "to reduce the number of inappropriate admissions of geriatric patients to state mental hospitals" (Screening Unit Memo #124, December 21, 1964). By referrals to other community resources and to home treatment, the unit has reduced substantially the number of commitments.

By the time of the first follow-up, patients were in various locations, and the research team had moved its offices from the General Hospital in San Francisco to the Langley Porter Neuropsychiatric Institute. Some patients had been discharged from the hospital directly to their homes in the community (17 per cent), others had been sent to private hospitals or rest homes (12 per cent), a small proportion of the patients had died while still in the hospital (3 per cent), more than two-thirds (68 per cent) had been sent to state hospitals. For our sample the odds were two to one that a person admitted to the General Hospital's psychiatric wards would later be admitted to a state hospital. By the time the staff attempted to interview the patients approximately one and two years later, the percentage of patients in institutions was reduced considerably, while the percentage of patients who died increased more than ten times.

If a patient discharged to the community from the screening wards went from his home to a nursing home, from the nursing home back to the screening wards, from there to a state hospital, where he stayed until he was seen at the time of follow-up, he was

| | Follow-up Interviews | |
| | First | Second |
Location status	Percentage	
Died	35	44
In state hospital	31	23
In other institutional facility	7	7
In community	24	23
Not located	3	3
N	(534)	(534)

counted simply as being in a state hospital, since he happened to be there at the time of the follow-up.

Because the possibilities for a normal existence are severely curtailed in a state hospital or other institutional setting, the questionnaires developed by the research staff for the initial interview were inappropriate for the later interviews, so two versions of each schedule administered by the social interviewers (who at the time of the follow-ups were also trained to administer the psychological rating instruments) were developed: one for those persons then living in the community, and one for those then in institutions. The questionnaires administered to the latter group of patients were limited to the areas of self-maintenance, psychological status, and interviewer ratings; while the questionnaires for those in the community covered, in addition, others pertaining to socioeconomic status, social interaction, leisure-time activities, and physical symptoms.

The project psychiatrist developed a medical schedule for follow-up interviewing, based on data modified from the baseline medical forms and the baseline health schedule. New data on reasons for continued hospitalization, state hospital and project psychiatrists' diagnoses, specific disabilities, specific geriatric problems, and treatment procedures were included. The research schedule used by the psychiatrists during the second follow-up was considerably more detailed than the earlier one. It repeated data previously covered and included objective check-lists for responses to each item in a mental status examination.

There was no attempt to obtain collateral information at the time of the follow-ups because it was felt that the research staff would be occupied entirely with interviewing patients. For this reason, the amount and reliability of information gathered at the follow-ups may be somewhat less than that obtained at baseline—especially for those patients who were in institutions.

The social interviewer-psychologists attempted to interview all survivors at each follow-up (65 per cent and 56 per cent, respectively, the first and second follow-ups). Because the psychiatric staff was too small to cover all survivors, it was decided at the first follow-up that the psychiatrists should try to interview all the patients in a state hospital and only those in the community who had been discharged or were on a leave of absence from a state hospital. At the second follow-up the psychiatrists' sample was expanded to include patients in other institutions, including those who went to these other institutions directly from the screening wards and those transferred from state hospitals. At the end of the data-collecting years, survivors from the original sample had been covered as follows:

	Follow-up	
	First	*Second*
	Percentage	
Social interviewer/psychologist and psychiatrist	50	52
Social interviewer/psychologist only	33	31
Psychiatrist only	1	1
Refused	4	6
Not seen (moved out of Bay Area or considered chronic not-at-home after three interview attempts)	8	5
Location unknown	4	5
N	(348)	(298)

In addition to the two follow-up rounds of interviewing, staff psychiatrists developed three supplemental schedules. To collect additional data about the physical and psychiatric condition of these patients during their stay on the general hospital screening wards, a staff psychiatrist conducted and supervised a detailed review of the San Francisco General Hospital psychiatric ward charts for all 534 cases in the original sample. (Langley Porter residents, working overtime, assisted him.) The main objective of this work was to collect data about treatment and course of illness that would provide a basis for making informed psychiatric judgments of the extent and nature of change in the patient's condition during the screening period. Concurrently, another staff psychiatrist supervised the completing of a research schedule for 230 patients who had died at state hospitals or other accessible institutions between the baseline and the first follow-up or between the first and second follow-ups. This schedule was to provide data on change in the patient's physical and psychiatric condition and to record causes of death. Then we reviewed the medical ward charts for approximately eighty patients who had been transferred from the psychiatric screening wards to the medical wards of the San Francisco General Hospital. All the research schedules used on the project throughout the three years of data collection are listed in Appendix B.

CHAPTER ONE

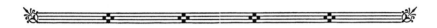

Background

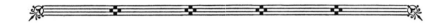

Except for a survey conducted by Vera Norris in London (Norris, 1959) that included some reference to geriatric admissions to mental hospitals, this inquiry—to the best of our knowledge—is the only large scale study of older mental patients who comprise a near-universe of patients in psychiatric screening or observation wards rather than in state hospitals.[1] Blau and his associates (Blau, Arth, Kettell, West, and Oppenheim, 1962; D. Blau, 1966) studied a much smaller group, with some remarkable similarities in findings. A study, in some ways growing out of the one reported here, is now being conducted in Harris County, Texas, by Charles M. Gaitz, Paul E. Baer, and associates. A significant difference, however, is that this study is a demonstration project offering care of suspected mentally ill aged. Although our extensive sampling procedure had a delimiting effect on the clinical follow-up (persons who returned

---

[1] Unfortunately, comparisons with the London material are virtually impossible because the age groupings for the older patients in that study are fifty to sixty-nine and seventy and over.

to the community directly from the general hospital and who were still residing there at the time of the second and third annual contacts could not be examined individually by psychiatrists), its advantages were twofold: it provided a borderline group between those committed to state hospitals and those living in the community, and it provided an opportunity to compare the condition of the patients at the time of admission to the screening wards with their condition at the time of disposition from the screening wards, an average of seven days later.

THE SCREENING WARD SAMPLE

The study sample consisted of 534 persons sixty years of age and older who were admitted to the San Francisco General Hospital psychiatric screening wards in 1959. The total number of persons in this age group admitted to these wards was 774, which represented approximately 17 per cent of all screening ward admissions during that year. This proportion was similar to that of persons aged sixty and older in the general population of San Francisco (18 per cent, according to 1960 U.S. census figures). The gross number of elderly admissions in 1959 represented a decrease over the fiscal years 1956–57 (841) and 1957–58 (879). Although the decrease might be ascribed to an official effort on the part of the California Department of Mental Hygiene to discourage the admission of so-called "harmless seniles," the evidence for such a conclusion is not very convincing. In the first place, nearly identical directives on this subject were issued during all three years. Secondly, since women seventy-five and older predominate among those having a diagnosis of chronic senile brain syndrome, one would expect that, if the decrease resulted from a policy of admitting fewer seniles, the very elderly would have been under-represented in 1959 compared with the earlier years. Actually, there were somewhat more women in the 1959 group than in the two preceding years, and the age distributions were almost identical.

The entire 774 elderly admissions in 1959 did not constitute the sample for the study because it was decided to maximize the possibility of focusing on age-linked mental disorders. All persons who had had psychiatric admissions before age sixty were excluded (63 per cent of the 240 ineligible), as were persons with a history of arrests prior to age sixty (2 per cent).[2] In addition, patients returned to the psychiatric ward after leaving a state hospital without permission or after failing to return when permitted to go on limited leave also were excluded (12 per cent), as were those who had not been county residents for at least a year (23 per cent), the latter on the assumption that they would be transferred to another state and therefore be difficult to include in follow-up studies. Nearly twice as many men as women were screened out of the sample for these reasons, and over half (52 per cent) of this ineligible group was under age sixty-five. As might be expected, in view of the screening criteria, there were proportionately more persons with psychogenic diagnoses or diagnoses of alcoholism among the ineligible than in the sample selected (neither of these disorders is as likely to have its inception in late life as is organic brain disorder). The same proportion of each group (two-thirds) was committed to state hospitals, but slightly more of the ineligible, mainly alcoholics, were discharged to the community, whereas more of the sample were discharged to medical or custodial institutions.

To develop an informed estimate of the extent to which this sample was representative of all elderly persons in San Francisco who were hospitalized for psychiatric reasons in 1959, a survey was made of private and public psychiatric institutions in the San Francisco Bay Area that were known to accept patients from San Francisco (California Department of Mental Hygiene, 1960b). In all, there were 114 admissions of elderly persons to such facilities during the study year. In other words, the 774 admissions to the San Francisco General Hospital psychiatric screening wards represented 87 per cent of all elderly persons in San Francisco who were admitted to psychiatric inpatient facilities in that year; the study sample represented 60 per cent of all such persons. The records kept at these other institutions did not indicate how many of the 114 persons had been admitted to psychiatric facilities prior to age sixty. The sex ratio of these other admissions was about equal, whereas in the screening ward sample and in that segment of it sent to state hospitals, there were proportionately a few more women than men.

---

[2] Only a selection of the tabular data on which this report is based is presented. Additional tables, listed in Appendix D, are available upon request.

Table 1

COMPARISON BETWEEN PROJECT SAMPLE AND
ADMISSIONS TO OTHER PSYCHIATRIC FACILITIES

	Total project sample	State hospitalized (from project sample)	Admissions to other psychiatric facilities
	Per cent	Per cent	Per cent
Male	47	46	49
Under 65	14	11	28
Married	22	22	56
Single	17	16	14
Separated or divorced	20	22	4
Protestant	40	41	41
Lived alone or in custodial institution	59	59	27
Medium or high Tryon score	29	30	54
Primary diagnosis psychogenic	20	17	59
Committed to state hospital	65	100	1
Less than one month stay	-	13	67
N	(534)	(348)	(114)

Persons admitted to other psychiatric facilities were younger than those in the study sample who were sent from the screening wards to state hospitals. Partly because of their age, the other admissions were more than twice as likely to be married as those in the study sample, although the proportion who were single was about the same. There were no notable religious differences between the two groups, but they differed markedly in social living arrangements, those admitted to other institutions being far less likely to have lived alone or to have lived in custodial institutions prior to admission than those who went to the screening wards of the general hospital. This is a reflection of the higher proportion of younger persons and of married persons among those admitted to other institutions.

No uniform data on socioeconomic status were collected by the other facilities canvassed, but by using the home addresses of patients and the census tract Index of Socioeconomic Independence developed for San Francisco by Tryon (1955), it was possible to make rough comparisons. As one might expect, inasmuch as several of the other facilities were private, the differences in socioeconomic status were marked: more than one-half of those admitted to other institutions were on a medium or high level of socioeconomic independence as measured by this index, while more than two-thirds of those in the sample were in the two lowest quartiles.

Differences in diagnosis also were striking: more than one-half (59 per cent) of the persons admitted to other institutions were diagnosed as having psychogenic disorders, 25 per cent had chronic brain syndromes, and only 7 per cent were assigned a diagnosis of acute brain syndrome. In the project sample, of the 525 who received diagnoses, 20 per cent were assigned a primary diagnosis of psychogenic disorder, 27 per cent of chronic brain syndrome, and more than one-half (53 per cent) were given diagnoses of acute brain syndrome. (Project diagnoses reported here are primary diagnoses, that is, those that, in the judgment of the project psychiatrist, were the cause of the patient's admission to the psychiatric ward. For a detailed analysis of the diagnostic terminology and procedures used, see Chapter Three.)

At first glance, one might conclude that elderly San Franciscans suffering from acute or chronic brain syndromes were likely to come from a low socioeconomic stratum and were therefore sent to a public rather than a private hospital. It indeed may be true that acute brain syndromes (frequently due to alcoholism or malnutrition or both) are a more common affliction in the lower socioeconomic groups, but there is no evidence in the epidemiological or clinical literature to suggest that this is true of chronic brain syndromes. An alternative explanation seems more likely, namely, that a large number of persons with chronic brain syndromes were being cared for in nursing homes or on the medical rather than psychiatric wards of private hospitals. And we know that about one per cent of the subjects in our community sample suffered from severe chronic brain disorders and were living, in effect, on one-person wards at home (Lowenthal et al., 1967).

The subsequent fate of the two groups of patients is difficult to compare precisely because of wide variations in record-keeping among the institutions surveyed. However, it is possible to say that at the time the records of other psychiatric inpatient facilities were reviewed (three to four years after the 1959 patients were admitted), 79 per cent of the patients under consideration had been released to the community, 12 per cent had been sent to other institutions (mainly nursing or old age homes), and 7 per cent had died while in residence. Two-thirds, furthermore, had stayed less than one month. The picture was dramatically different for the state hospitalized patients in the project sample, of whom, approximately two years after admission, 23 per cent were in the community, 23 per cent were still in a state hospital, and nearly one-half (44 per cent) were dead. In view of the younger age level and the preponderance of psychogenic disorders among those admitted to other institutions, and the preponderance of acute brain syndromes and physical illnesses among the project sample, these differences are not surprising. Had these privately hospitalized patients been sent to the San Francisco General Hospital psychiatric ward, the impact on the project sample would have been relatively slight as most of them no doubt would have been screened out because of psychiatric admissions prior to age sixty. On the basis of this assumption, we believe it a reasonable estimate that the sample studied represented between 90 and 95 per cent of all elderly psychiatric *first* admissions from San Francisco in 1959. It is, in short, a cohort of those urban aged who in a given year are likely to need, for the first time in their lives, psychiatric attention at a time of crisis.

SAN FRANCISCO'S ELDERLY

There were few differences of sex and nativity (born in California, elsewhere in the United States, or in foreign countries), between the screening ward sample and the elderly population of San Francisco as a whole. About one-fourth of each group was born in California, and over one-third (36 per cent) of each was born abroad. There is little support, with this age group, for the hypothesis of a relation between geographic mobility and mental illness. Compared with elderly San Franciscans as a whole, Caucasians were very slightly over-represented among the hospitalized, while most other races were slightly under-represented. Orientals, not differentiated in census data, were estimated to be considerably under-represented, a matter that the project staff hopes eventually to make the object of systematic inquiry. There were relatively few Negroes, reflecting the comparative youthfulness of the Negro population of San Francisco.

The very old were considerably over-represented among those hospitalized on the screening wards, 26 per cent being eighty years or older, compared with 10 per cent (among persons sixty and older) in the population at large. Conversely, younger people were under-represented: 14 per cent of the hospitalized were between sixty and sixty-four, compared with 32 per cent of the older population of San Francisco. Although the ratio of men to women was about the same for the hospitalized as for elderly San Franciscans (the hospital sample was 47 per cent male, the elderly of San Francisco 46 per cent), there were notable age differences within the two sex groups. Patients between the ages of sixty and sixty-four were under-represented in the hospital sample for both sex groups, but this was more true of women than of men (among whom there were more alcoholics, who were generally under seventy). Among persons seventy-five years of age and older, the sex differences were most notable: one-fourth of the elderly women of San Francisco were seventy-five or older, whereas more than half (55 per cent) of the women in the screening ward sample fell into this age group. Twenty per cent of the elderly men of San Francisco were seventy-five and older, while 36 per cent of the hospitalized men fell into this age group. It should be noted that the elderly of San Francisco closely resemble the elderly of California and of the United States as a whole in the age distribution of both men and women. As a result, in part, of this high proportion of older women in the sample, the group reaching the screening wards in San Francisco included considerably fewer married persons than did older San Franciscans in general (22 per cent, compared with 44 per cent), and more who were widowed (39 per cent, compared with 31 per cent). Proportionately twice as many of the hospitalized as of the elderly population in general were separated or divorced. The proportion of single persons (17 per cent, compared with 15 per cent), however, was similar to that in the elderly population at large.

Those who reached the psychiatric wards were far more likely to be retired than were their counterparts in the community: 91 per cent were retired, compared with 66 per cent of their non-institutionalized cohorts. This discrepancy between the hospitalized and those in the community held at each age level: 80 per cent of the hospitalized males who were between sixty and sixty-four were retired or unemployed, compared with an estimated 17 per cent in the country as a whole (Seidner, 1960) and 26 per cent in San Francisco (1960 census). The hospitalized had been retired longer than elderly San Franciscans in general, as might be expected from their greater age. In view of their lower employment rate, it is not surprising that the screening ward group had a considerably lower socioeconomic status than that of their age cohorts in the community. Census and project data were not strictly comparable because the census question pertained to individual income (thus a wife supported by her husband would be recorded as having no income), whereas the project question covered the income of the subject and his or her spouse if they lived in the same dwelling unit. Even so, the hospitalized were considerably poorer than elderly San Franciscans in general. Omitting persons who had no income, on the grounds that these were largely wives (with a scattering of persons living in and supported by households of adult children), the census data show that 59 per cent of elderly San Franciscans had annual incomes of under $2,000, compared with 70 per cent of the hospital sample. Conversely, only 11 per cent of the hospital sample had annual incomes of $3,000 or more compared with 25 per cent in the community at large.

The hospitalized were distinguished by considerably more residential (rather than geographic) mobility than were their counterparts in the community: more than one-half (52 per cent) had moved within the past five years, compared with slightly more than one-third (35 per cent) of elderly San Franciscans in general. This discrepancy was only partly accounted for by moves to nursing or old age homes because of illnesses that they had had, often for a long time, before they were admitted to the psychiatric wards. Many elderly persons who were suffering from psychogenic disorders, including alcoholism, had moved several times in the year prior to psychiatric ward admission. Often the moves could be interpreted as symptoms of illness. Those who were hospitalized were considerably more likely to have been living alone than were elderly San Franciscans in general. Census data are available only for those who are sixty-five and older, but, within this age group, 34 per cent of the aged living in the community compared with 46 per cent of those sixty-five and older in our hospitalized group, lived alone. (For analyses of isolation, mental illness, and treatment for mental illness in old age, see Lowenthal, 1964b, 1966.)

SCREENING WARD SAMPLE AND A MATCHED SUBSAMPLE

The project hospitalized sample differed from the elderly of San Francisco particularly in their marital and employment status and residential mobility. To answer the question of whether these characteristics resulted from the greater age, poverty, and preponderance of older women among the hospitalized and to compare levels of functioning between the aged living in the community and those who were hospitalized, subsamples of 268 persons from each of the community and hospital samples were matched for age, sex, and socioeconomic status. These subsamples were older and poorer than their counterparts age sixty and older in San Francisco and included somewhat more men, 51 per cent, than the 46 per cent in the community as a whole.

Contrary to expectations stemming from studies of psychiatric hospitalization of all age groups (for example, Kramer, Taube and Starr, 1968), we found proportionately fewer single and more married persons among the hospitalized than among the nonhospitalized subsamples. This was partly a result of the stratified sampling procedure used in the community (over-sampling men who live alone). The proportion that was separated or divorced, however, conformed with expectations: 21 per cent of the hospitalized, compared with 16 per cent of the community subsample, fell into one of these categories. The proportion that was divorced was about the same, most of the discrepancy being accounted for by the higher proportion of hospitalized subjects who were separated. Even though the two groups were matched for age, sex, and socioeconomic status, the proportion that was employed was considerably higher in the community subsample (21 per cent, compared with 6 per cent). One-half of the hospitalized sample, compared with 40 per cent of the nonhospitalized, had moved within the preceding five years, and proportionately twice as many hospitalized patients had moved within the previous year (25 per cent, compared with 13 per cent).

Comparative data for a few social characteristics noted in the matched subsamples are not available for the San Francisco population in general. The married among the two subsample groups were about as likely to have children (59 per cent of the hospitalized and 60 per cent of the nonhospitalized), the hospitalized were slightly more likely to have children living in the Bay Area (49 and 46 per cent, respectively); those in the community subsample were more likely to live alone than those in the hospitalized subsample (60 per cent, compared with 44 per cent). However, this last variable was controlled for the community group: ten per cent of the hospitalized subsample had lived in institutions before being admitted to the screening wards, most of them in nursing homes or the county old age home, whereas persons currently in institutions were deliberately excluded from the community sample. The hospitalized were less likely to live in apartments or hotels and more likely to live in their own homes. This was no doubt an artifact of the sampling procedures used in the community: the census tracts with the highest proportion of elderly persons also have the highest proportion of rental units; their living alone was a screening criterion for half of the community sample; and people who live alone are more likely to live in rental units than in their own homes. According to the 1960 census, about one-half of the elderly of San Francisco as a whole own their homes, but only 17 per cent of our hospitalized and 5 per cent of our nonhospitalized samples did so. These discrepancies are partly the result of higher proportions, in both samples, of the very old who are more likely to live alone. There were somewhat more Catholics among the hospitalized, while the community subjects were more likely to report no religious affiliation. The hospitalized subjects tended to have lived in the city slightly longer than the nonhospitalized, but in this there were no appreciable differences.

On an index of physical disability,[3] 40 per cent of the hospitalized, compared with 2 per cent of the community group, ranked as severely disabled; 19 per cent of the latter group had no physical disability, whereas all of the hospital subsample were disabled. The hospitalized were more than twice as likely to have been in hospital for physical reasons at least three times during the past ten years as were community subsample subjects, and, conversely, they were less likely not to have been in hospital at all (24 per cent, compared with 43 per cent). The hospitalized subjects were about three times as likely to have suffered from a stroke and half again as likely to have reported heart disorders in the past year as were the community subjects. Few differences in other health problems or diseases were noticed, except that the community subsample reported more fractures and more kidney ailments in the past ten years than did the hospitalized subsample. On the basis of interviewer ratings, only a few more of the hospitalized appeared to suffer from hearing disabilities. Unfortunately, no strictly comparable data were available on eyesight as the community sample assessed their own visual defects (26 per cent reported problems) while, in the hospital sample, the physician rated vision (15 per cent with problems). The most telling indication of the difference in health between the two groups, however, was mortality. Within six months of the initial contact, 25 per cent of the hospitalized subsample were dead, compared with less than 3 per cent of the community subsample. At the end of two years, 44 per cent of the hospitalized subsample had died, compared with 9 per cent of the community subsample.

Those in the hospitalized group were far more psychiatrically disturbed than those in the community subsample. Eighty-five per cent of those in hospital were rated as being severely disturbed and in need of full-time psychiatric supervision at the time of admission, in the judgment of the project psychiatrists. Project psychiatrists also rated community subjects from their protocols, and, by these

---

[3] This index is based on four measures of health: major physical illness in the past ten years, two or more days in bed at home during the past year, a visit to a physician or clinic in the past month, and two or more days in the hospital during the past year.

procedures, 7 per cent of the community subsample was considered severely disabled. (For a comparison of social, physical, and psychiatric differences between the psychiatrically impaired in the community sample and the hospitalized, see Lowenthal et al., 1967). Also, even though persons who had been admitted to psychiatric institutions before the age of sixty were excluded from the sample, 37 per cent reported that they had been to a physician or clinic for "nerves" at some time in their lives, compared with only 13 per cent in the community subgroup. In addition to various indicators of psychiatric disability, a list of nine symptoms considered to be stereotypical indicators of a normal aging process was included in the protocol.[4] Nearly four times as many of the hospitalized had five or more such symptoms, although for them, the questions were answered on the basis of "best available data" and included information from relatives, while community subjects answered for themselves.

In view of the considerable mental and physical discrepancies, it was not surprising to find that the hospitalized were functioning on considerably lower levels than were the nonhospitalized. Measured against functional levels of self-maintenance—dressing, safety, feeding, locomotion, going to the toilet, and money management—almost all of the community subsample were completely independent, whereas most of the hospitalized needed some assistance or supervision during the period just prior to admission. Discrepancies in the level of social interaction were equally dramatic. Judged on an index of current role status, which included the roles of spouse, parent, church member, organization member, and employment, the current role status of the two groups was similar, but the level of social interaction of the hospitalized was considerably lower: in the two weeks prior to admission, almost half of them had had contacts only with persons in their dwelling unit, or with shopkeepers or persons met casually in a park or cafeteria, while little more than one-tenth of the community subsample had had as restricted social contacts.

---

[4] These symptoms are a reduction or loss of energy, memory, interest in personal appearance, or appetite; increases in irritability, being bothered by little things or worried for no reason at all; tendencies to lose or misplace objects; erratic spirits.

COMPARISONS BETWEEN LOS ANGELES AND SAN FRANCISCO

More than two-thirds of the screening ward patients, 68 per cent, were committed directly to state hospitals after court hearings on the psychiatric wards, 17 per cent were discharged to the community, the remainder were sent to other institutions such as medical hospitals and the county old age home (12 per cent), or died on the psychiatric screening wards (3 per cent).

Some fairly comparable data from other parts of the country are available on patients committed to state hospitals. San Francisco has long been singled out for its high rates of a variety of disorders such as mental illness commitment rates, alcoholism, and suicide. Customarily, comparisons between San Francisco and Los Angeles are comparisons between the two counties. The differences shown in such comparisons are dramatic: in 1959, the commitment rate of persons sixty and older (first admissions), was four hundred per one hundred thousand for San Francisco compared with ninety-four per one hundred thousand for Los Angeles.[5] On the face of it, such comparisons might be misleading, because, while the 44.6 square miles of the city and county of San Francisco are consolidated and almost completely urbanized, the 4,060 square miles of Los Angeles county includes suburban and rural districts. However, tables separating the city of Los Angeles from the county revealed few differences: the commitment rate of the city elderly (one hundred and one per one hundred thousand) was similar to that of the county. Therefore, we followed custom and compared the two counties. In the age, sex, and educational distribution of the population age 60 and over, Los Angeles and San Francisco counties closely resembled each other, although Los Angeles county had fewer persons sixty and older (13 per cent) than did San Francisco county (18 per cent). However, the distribution of persons from the two counties admitted to state hospitals in 1959 (excluding those with

[5] The differences held for all age groups; the overall rate for Los Angeles is ninety-one per one hundred thousand and for San Francisco three hundred and sixty per one hundred thousand (California Department of Mental Hygiene, 1960a). Incidentally, the city of San Francisco occupies the entire area of the county of San Francisco.

psychiatric admissions before age sixty)[6] differed rather noticeably. In comparison with the elderly population of the county, the hospitalized San Franciscans considerably over-represented persons eighty and older and considerably under-represented those under sixty-five, whereas the Los Angeles hospitalized more closely followed the age distribution for the county as a whole.

Discrepancies were even more marked in the age distribution within each sex. In the screening ward sample, older San Francisco women were considerably over-represented when compared with older San Francisco men. When those sent to state hospitals from San Francisco were compared with those sent from Los Angeles in the same period, the differences were considerable. In Los Angeles, the aged distribution of both committed men and women closely resembled the age distribution of the elderly population in general. In San Francisco, more than one-half of the committed women were seventy-five or older, whereas only one-fourth of the elderly female population was; among men the differences were not as extreme. In Los Angeles county, there were no differences in the proportions of older women and older men committed. As for similarly dispro- portionate rates of alcoholism and mental illness in all age groups, the usual explanation for these discrepancies is that there are many more alternative facilities for the care of such problems in Los An- geles than in San Francisco. At the end of 1959, for example, there were few more nursing and convalescent homes per 100,000 persons aged sixty and older in Los Angeles than there were in San Fran- cisco, but there were two and one-half times as many beds. Private institutions specifically licensed for the care of mentally ill geriatric patients were even more numerous: in July 1959 in Los Angeles there were nine institutions and 458 beds per 100,000 persons sixty and over; in San Francisco there were three institutions and thirteen beds per 100,000. One reasonable explanation for the dispropor- tionate number of older women admitted in San Francisco might be that, since older men are more likely to be married and therefore

[6] Data summarized here were made available by the Biostatistics Section, California Department of Mental Hygiene. The total number of San Franciscans in the state tabulations exceeds the total number of patients in state hospitals who comprised the project sample because the former number includes transfers from hospitals and probably some nonresidents.

Table 2

Los Angeles and San Francisco Counties: Comparisons of Elderly Population in General With Those in State Hospitals

	Los Angeles		San Francisco	
	Total age 60+ Population	State Hospitalized	Total age 60+ Population	State Hospitalized
	Per cent	Per cent	Per cent	Per cent
Under 65	30	29	32	20
80 or older	11	12	10	23
Male	42	48	46	50
Some high school at least	43	32	41	35
Caucasian	95	91	93	97
Married	51	42	44	24
Divorced or separated	8	19	10	15
Single	8	9	15	20

to have someone to take care of them at home, it is the very elderly women who benefit most from the more plentiful nursing homes available in Los Angeles.[7]

From Table 2, we see that the poorly educated who were in hospital were slightly more over-represented in Los Angeles than in San Francisco. San Francisco county had slightly fewer elderly Negroes and more patients of other races than did Los Angeles and, whereas the elderly hospitalized from Los Angeles under-represented the elderly Caucasians in the county as a whole and over-represented persons from other races, the trend was just the opposite in San Francisco. In San Francisco the proportion of single elderly persons was almost twice as large as in Los Angeles—and these were over-represented among the hospitalized in San Francisco— whereas in Los Angeles the hospitalized and nonhospitalized resembled each other. In both counties, the divorced and separated were over-represented; the married, among those hospitalized, were under-represented.

COMPARISONS WITH CALIFORNIA AND OTHER STATES

In comparison with elderly patients admitted to state hospitals throughout California (California Department of Mental Hygiene, 1960a), those sent to state hospitals from the project sample were slightly better educated, older, and proportionately more were women (see Table 1).[8] Comparable data for the states of New York (Malzberg, 1956) and Ohio (Locke, Kramer, and Pasamanick, 1960) revealed no consistent patterns. However, the dates of the studies varied considerably. The ages of the state hospital patients in the San Francisco sample were more similar to the state hospital patients in New York and Ohio than to those in California as a whole, where more patients are under seventy-five. Sex distribution followed a similar pattern: the San Francisco sample and that of New York State had more women than men; California had

---

[7] In the country as a whole, 58 per cent of the men who are seventy-five or older are married, compared to 21 per cent of the women in the same age group (Sheldon, 1963). Comparable figures for the screening ward sample studied are 24 per cent and 6 per cent respectively.

[8] The Department of Mental Hygiene data are for persons sixty-five and over, the usual cutting off point for state hospital statistics.

Table 3

Comparisons of Project Sample, California, and Other States (Patients Sixty-Five and Older)

	State Hospitalized From Project Sample (1959) Per cent	Ohio[a] (1948–1952) Per cent	California[b] (1959) Per cent	New York[c] (1948) Per cent	Kansas[d] (1956) Per cent	United States Average[d] Per cent
Deceased within one year	38	-	34	45	27	-
Some high school at least	26	-	23	-	-	-
75 or older	56	53	45	52	-	-
Male	44	55	50	45	-	-
Caucasian	97	93	93	96	-	-
Discharged within one year	18	-	28	11[e]	45	-
Diseases of the senium[f]	75	-	77	-	-	83
N	(309)	(4,710)	(3,154)	(5,122)	(306)	(33,485)

[a] Locke, Kramer, and Pasamanick, 1960.
[b] California Department of Mental Hygiene, 1960a.
[c] Malzberg, 1956.
[d] Pollack, Locke, and Kramer, 1961.
[e] United States Public Health Service, 1959.
[f] Mainly cerebral arteriosclerosis and senile brain disease.

equal numbers; Ohio had 45 per cent women, 55 per cent men. The project state hospitalized sample included fewer nonwhites than appear in California first admissions in general and, again, the project sample looked rather like New York State in this respect (since the New York State figures were for 1948, subsequent population shifts may have altered the ratios). Differences in the dates of these studies may well present even greater problems when it comes to location after one year: the state hospitalized in the project sample (1959) were somewhat more likely to be deceased (38 per cent) and considerably less likely to be in the community (18 per cent) a year after admission than were California elderly first admissions as a whole (34 and 28 per cent, respectively, in 1953–1954). New York State (1953–1954) had a poorer showing than California or the project sample in this respect, whereas Kansas (1956) reported a phenomenal 45 per cent in the community and only 27 per cent deceased. These discrepancies are impossible to interpret, since comparable data were not available for age distributions, diagnosis, and admission, treatment, and discharge policies. In fact, the only diagnostic comparisons possible were between the project state hospitalized group, Calfornia, and the United States average based on a survey in eleven states for the period 1954–58 (Pollack, Locke, and Kramer, 1961). Even here, data collecting practices permitted comparison of only two general diagnostic categories: diseases of the senium (cerebral arteriosclerosis and senile brain disease) and schizophrenic reactions. The figures for those sent to state hospitals from the project sample and for all California admissions for the same year showed proportionately fewer in the category of diseases of the senium and more in the "all over" (which includes acute brain syndrome, affective disorders, and alcohol addiction) than the average for the United States as a whole. It will be recalled that sample subjects were given multiple diagnoses by project psychiatrists, but in this context only the diagnosis considered as the main reason for admission, the primary diagnosis, was used.

SUMMARY

The screening ward sample differed from the universe of elderly San Franciscans from which it was drawn in being older and in including proportionately more women than men age seventy-five and older, fewer married persons, somewhat fewer Negroes, and considerably fewer Orientals. Even those age sixty to sixty-four were far less likely to have been employed than were their counterparts in the community, and their socioeconomic status, indicated by their annual income, was far lower. They were more likely to have been living alone. Persons discharged from the screening wards to the community more closely resembled the elderly population as a whole on these counts than did persons committed to state mental hospitals.

Subsamples matched for age, sex, and socioeconomic status were drawn from the two project samples. The hospitalized included somewhat more divorced or separated and more married persons than did the community group, and they also showed far more residential mobility. The community subsample included many more employed persons, but otherwise the hospitalized showed fewer symptoms of social disintegration than one might expect: they were more likely to have children in the Bay Area, more likely to have a religious affiliation, and more likely to own their homes than was the community subsample. They were, however, in far worse physical condition than their community counterparts and, ranked far lower according to measures of self-maintenance and social interaction.

Because of the stratified nature of the community sample (over-sampling of persons living alone), it would be unwise to draw conclusions about marital status. However, according to other measures of social integration, the elderly who were hospitalized for mental illness did not differ greatly from their community counterparts, except in factors that their illness might affect, such as unemployment, residential mobility, and a low level of social interaction. By far the most dramatic distinguishing characteristic of those who were hospitalized was their very poor physical condition and accompanying difficulties in self-maintenance.

In San Francisco, a far higher proportion of the elderly arrived at state hospitals in 1959 than in Los Angeles, principally because Los Angeles has more alternative facilities. In comparison with the Los Angeles hospitalized, the San Francisco group included proportionately more women seventy-five or older, and non-

Caucasians were under-represented. Compared with elderly first admissions in the state as a whole, the project sample had proportionately more women, more older persons, and more Caucasians; educational background was similar in the two groups. Elderly first admissions in California as a whole differed from those of other states for which data were available, but no patterns were discernible.

Partly as a result of previously reported findings from this research, the California Department of Mental Hygiene established in October, 1963, a Geriatric Screening Unit at the San Francisco General Hospital to evaluate elderly psychiatric patients and to seek alternatives to state hospitalization. The staff, a psychiatrist, an internist, and two social workers, in two years, reduced state hospital admissions among persons sixty and over from an average of forty-two per month to an average of two per month. In 1967, only three patients were committed; up to May 1968, only two. The four professionals on this team have been able to see patients in their homes, thus forestalling their arrival on the screening wards, and to search out alternative arrangements for their care—time-consuming tasks that could not have been managed by the limited regular staff of the screening wards. In February, 1966, the Langley Porter geriatric research group received a small grant from the California Department of Mental Hygiene to follow-up the patients for whom the screening team is now finding other solutions and to compare their progress with that of patients committed to state hospitals in 1959 and followed-up in the course of the research reported in this volume (Epstein and Simon, 1968).

In view of the remarkable success of the geriatric screening team in preventing state hospital admissions of the elderly, it might well be asked whether the practical objectives of our own research have not thus been achieved, and why it is necessary to analyze our study sample in such detail. The answers provide one of the major objectives of this book. The group of 534 persons has been studied in greater detail, to the best of our knowledge, than has any other large group of elderly mental patients. Although the achievements of the screening team have been nothing short of astonishing we suspect that the alternative arrangements for care are far from adequate, and will soon become overtaxed. One of the challenges confronting the Medicare program will be to provide satisfactory comprehensive treatment and care for the mentally ill aged. This book aims to describe in detail the nature and course of the mental illness of a group of elderly city-dwellers who are representative of those who will seek or require aid for psychiatric disturbances in any given year.

CHAPTER TWO

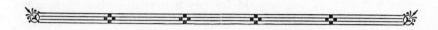

Post-Admission
Assessment

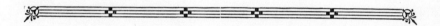

Two assumptions commonly held about the admission of an elderly person to a mental hospital are that he has lost most of his social and economic supports and that he is being shunted off by children or community agencies unwilling to expend any effort on his care. These assumptions were explored in *Lives in Distress* (Lowenthal, 1964a) by analyzing the decisions in the admission to psychiatric screening wards of 530 of the 534 persons comprising the project hospital sample. The objectives of that study were to describe the social contexts in which such decision making takes place, to explore the attitudes of family and community toward psychopathologic manifestations among the elderly, and to develop insights into prevailing concepts of social responsibility for the mentally disturbed aged.

The patients, older, financially poorer, and physically sicker than those we studied in the community at large, were also more isolated socially. About one-tenth of them were true social isolates, without friends or relatives anywhere, and about the same proportion were semi-isolates, that is, their friends or relatives, for geographical or other reasons, were not available at the time of crisis. During the period just before hospitalization or immediately after it, four-fifths of all patients had relatives or friends who served either as decision makers or were informants to the research team or both.

In the analysis of reasons for hospitalization offered by relatives, friends, or other informants, the three most striking findings were that very few patients, in fact only 4 per cent, were reported to have had symptoms or problems in only one of five major categories (disturbances of thought or feeling, harmful or potentially harmful behavior, physical health, and environmental considerations), and nearly half had problems in four or in all five areas; that nearly three-fourths had at least one physical illness, disability, or symptom that was linked by the informant to admission; and that the predisposing factors had prevailed for some time: in one-third of the patients for five years or more, and in two-thirds for at least a year. Both the variety and duration of the predisposing and long-range conditions were more closely related to the fate of the patient than was the nature of the precipitating condition,[1] or such characteristics as socioeconomic status or degree of isolation. Unlike studies of younger patients, this analysis, primarily of reports from laymen, found relatively few examples of social or psychological trauma immediately preceding admission. Most of the patients had retired, lost a spouse, or suffered from physical illness or disability, but for the most part these changes had taken place in the distant past, often more than ten years prior to the patient's arrival on the psychiatric screening wards.

Analysis of the decision-making process showed that one-half of these patients had had arrangements made for their care before the precipitating symptom or circumstance developed, and nearly

[1] The precipitating condition was defined as the factor that triggered the first in a chain of events that ultimately led to the psychiatric ward. Predisposing factors were conditions insufficient in themselves to set off the chain of actions leading to the psychiatric ward, but considered by informants to be causally linked with the precipitant.

one-third of them had experienced two or more such alternatives. Most common were arrangements for additional support: a relative would be brought in or the patient would be moved to a nursing home or to the medical ward of a public or private hospital. About one-half of the arrangements had been in effect for six months or more and nearly one-fifth had lasted for at least three years. For an additional 10 per cent, alternatives were attempted but did not materialize because the patient refused to cooperate or because the nursing home or county old age home could or would not accept him. Steps taken after the development of the precipitant included requests for help or advice from relatives or physicians, examination of the patient by a physician, and the movement of the patient. For nearly two-thirds of the sample, at least three steps had been taken between the development of the precipitant and the admission to the psychiatric ward. Only 12 per cent were sent immediately to the psychiatric ward after the development of the precipitant. Most people who took the first step clearly did not have the psychiatric ward in mind at the time.

On an average, three persons were involved in the decisions for each patient, and, for most patients, at least one was a relative and one a physician. Usually, a private or public physician recommended admission to the psychiatric ward. Prevailing stereotypes to the contrary, very few landlords or relatives called for a police officer or an ambulance as soon as an acute situation developed. Police officers were involved at some point in 17 per cent of the cases, but they made the decision for the psychiatric ward in only 4 per cent. Self-admitted or voluntary patients, of whom there were thirty-six (7 per cent) generally had the fewest people involved in admission procedures. Even after the patient was admitted to the ward, relatives considered state hospitalization as the most realistic outcome in only one-half of the cases and as a preferred solution in only one-fifth—a striking contrast to the project psychiatrists' finding that 87 per cent of these patients were in need of full-time psychiatric care at the time of admission.[2]

[2] Research into reasons for the psychiatric hospitalization of the elderly at Boston State Hospital offer good support for the findings reported here. Reaffirming our conclusions, the study showed that family disinterest or neglect (the railroading so often suspected in such cases) were

PSYCHIATRIC ASSESSMENT

As soon as possible after subjects had been admitted to the screening wards, a research team of psychiatrists, psychologists, and social researchers interviewed and examined them. Very detailed information was recorded, including that furnished by collateral informants. The impairment, the functional level, and the resources of these patients were reported in terms of four domains: psychiatric status, physical status, self-maintenance, and certain psychosocial supports and deprivations.

Impairment ratings. After the psychiatric examinations, staff psychiatrists reviewed all other available information (see Appendix B for a list of the research schedules) and then rated each patient in the several categories commonly used to assess mental status. Combining all these data, they rated the over-all degree of psychiatric impairment for each patient. The global ratings generally coincided with the lowest rating the patient had received in any one of the nine mental status categories mentioned by Lowenthal and Berkman (1964). To simplify the reporting here, only the global ratings are used.

At the time of their admission, 87 per cent of the elderly patients were rated as being severely impaired, that is, in need of twenty-four-hour supervision. The remaining 13 per cent were rated as moderately impaired, that is, in need of considerable care or supervision, though not necessarily around-the-clock. Older subjects were no more likely to be severely impaired than were younger; in fact, proportionately more patients in their sixties were judged to be severely impaired than those in their eighties or older. Women were somewhat more likely to be severely impaired, but the sex differences were slight: 89 per cent, compared with 85 per cent. Women in the middle age range (seventy to seventy-nine) were

---

not significant factors in the sample of forty elderly psychiatric admissions (Arth, West, Blau, and Kettell, 1961); that physicians played the principal role in referring the patients to the psychiatric ward (D. Blau, 1961, 1966); that patients' behavior just prior to hospitalization—often presenting management or self-care problems as well as violently assaultive or self-destructive behavior—were crucial factors precipitating the hospitalization; and that psychopathological symptoms had been present for long periods before the patients' psychiatric admissions (Blau et al., 1962).

more severely impaired than were either the younger or the older women, and they were also more severely impaired than were men in the same age group.

During the pretest period the condition of many patients changed during their brief stay on the screening wards, but attempts to rate such change on the basis of a second psychiatric examination proved abortive because of the unpredictable and often very heavy case load of newly admitted patients who had to be examined as soon as possible. A team of project psychiatrists did return to the screening wards, after the baseline data had been collected, to review all the information in the hospital case files. Without referring to the initial rating, given when the patients were first admitted, the psychiatrists assigned "change on ward" ratings for each patient, for both physical and mental status. Eighteen per cent of the patients improved during their screening ward stay (an average of seven days), and 5 per cent deteriorated. Both age and sex made a difference in the likelihood for change. Nearly a third of those under seventy improved, while only 3 per cent of those eighty or older did so. Conversely, though far less dramatically, older patients were more likely to deteriorate. Men were more likely to improve than were women, but also they were more likely to deteriorate. These sex differences no doubt are partly the result of the greater frequency of acute brain syndrome among men, a condition that is by definition temporary and reversible if the underlying physical condition is not fatal.

Diagnosis. Multiple diagnoses permitted project psychiatrists to assign up to three psychiatric diagnoses for each patient, if warranted. The primary diagnosis was the condition that, in the psychiatrists' judgment, precipitated admission to the screening wards. The precipitating condition for more than half (53 per cent) of the 525 patients for whom it was possible to assign such diagnoses was acute brain syndrome, of which the most frequent physical causes were, in rank order: malnutrition, congestive heart failure, and acute or chronic alcoholism. The two other principal categories of precipitating condition were chronic brain syndrome (27 per cent) and psychogenic illness (20 per cent), of which depression was the most frequent. Twenty-six patients had attempted suicide just prior to admission, and about half of these had a primary diagnosis of acute brain syndrome, attributed mainly to the ingestion of sleeping pills. The other half were diagnosed as having psychogenic disorders, primarily depressions. Men were more likely to have an acute brain syndrome as a precipitant than women (60 versus 47 per cent), and in both sexes this diagnosis tended to increase with age. The increase with age was more strongly evident for chronic brain syndrome associated with arteriosclerosis or senility, and the increase was sharper for women: only 26 per cent of the oldest men had this disorder as precipitant, compared to 44 per cent of the oldest women. Psychogenic disorders were more prevalent among the youngest patients, particularly the women, and negligible among those eighty or older. Despite the high frequency of alcoholism in this sample (32 per cent among men, 15 per cent among women), alcoholism occurred as a sole precipitant, that is, without allied acute or chronic brain syndromes, in only 2 per cent of the sample.

Precipitant aside, when all the diagnoses assigned to each patient were considered, combinations were abundant, but five dominant groupings emerged. Fifty-four per cent of the patients showed organic brain syndrome, chronic or acute, but with no accompanying diagnosis of alcoholism or psychogenic disorder; 23 per cent showed alcoholism with or without brain syndrome; 9 per cent showed psychogenic disorders other than alcoholism and without brain syndrome; 10 per cent showed organic brain disorder and psychogenic disorder other than alcoholism; and 4 per cent showed chronic brain syndrome associated with causes other than senile or arteriosclerotic brain disease. Relatively few of the youngest, but 86 per cent of the oldest, patients were found in the first group. Nearly half of those in their sixties were in the alcoholism category, but few of the oldest appear here. Also, twice as many men as women were in this category.

However, as illuminating as these groupings might be, they are too numerous and cumbersome for analyzing the multitude of variables we are investigating here. Several substudies of the project (Trier, 1966, 1968; Epstein and Simon, 1969) have established that the presence of a psychogenic disorder in any diagnostic set is more crucial to the fate of the patient than is the nature of the precipitant itself or the degree of initial impairment. Accordingly,

Table 4

Psychiatric Status Indicators by Age and Sex

Psychiatric Domain	Men			Women			Total	
	60–69	70–79	80+	60–69	70–79	80+	Men	Women
	%	%	%	%	%	%	%	%
Impairment								
Moderate	13	16	16	10	6	17	15	11
Severe	87	84	84	90	94	83	85	89
N	(83)	(96)	(42)	(69)	(103)	(88)	(221)	(260)
Change on ward								
Improved	35	18	2	29	14	2	21	14
Unchanged	59	74	88	70	83	93	71	83
Deteriorated	6	8	10	1	3	5	8	3
N	(83)	(96)	(42)	(69)	(103)	(88)	(221)	(260)
Precipitating condition								
Acute brain syndrome	55	61	70	39	49	51	60	47
Chronic brain syndrome	15	24	26	18	33	44	21	33

	30	15	4	43	18	5	19	20
Psychogenic								
N	(94)	(107)	(46)	(74)	(107)	(97)	(247)	(278)
Psychogenic/Organic dichotomy								
Any psychogenic	73	46	13	75	30	12	49	36
Organic only[a]	27	54	87	25	70	88	51	64
N	(88)	(101)	(46)	(72)	(104)	(94)	(235)	(270)
Psychopathological symptoms								
None or 1	24	23	19	16	15	11	23	14
2 or 3	31	24	34	38	29	24	28	30
4 or 5	20	23	19	22	22	28	21	24
6 or more	25	30	28	24	34	37	28	32
N	(80)	(98)	(43)	(69)	(103)	(90)	(221)	(262)
Orientation								
in 3 spheres	46	21	12	49	16	8	29	22
in 2 spheres	19	23	15	11	18	14	20	15
in 1 sphere or none	27	40	41	31	50	64	35	50
Inaccessible	8	16	32	9	16	14	16	13
N	(88)	(98)	(41)	(70)	(104)	(90)	(227)	(264)

[a] Throughout volume, excludes "pure" acute brain syndrome.

in most of the subsequent analyses we use the following dichotomy: psychogenic disorder with or without accompanying acute or chronic brain syndrome (42 per cent, including alcoholics); and chronic brain syndrome, uncomplicated by psychogenic illness (58 per cent). In this dichotomy, however, we reduced the sample to 505, omitting those suffering from acute brain syndrome only (N = 20). It will be recalled that nine patients were not diagnosed. The presence of any psychogenic disorder within a set of multiple diagnoses decreased dramatically with age from nearly three-quarters of the youngest to somewhat more than one-tenth of the oldest. Sex differences were slight for the youngest and oldest, but within our middle age group, seventy to seventy-nine, these differences were marked. The large number of male alcoholics were no doubt swelling the ranks of the psychogenics.

Symptomatology. Reports of symptoms from the patient himself or his collateral provided another dimension of psychiatric condition. We had earlier learned, in comparing sixteen questions asked of both hospital and community sample subjects, that the number and type of reported symptoms had some relevance to psychiatric status (Lowenthal et al., 1967). We asked fourteen questions relating to psychopathological symptoms. Positive responses are listed in rank order and grouped according to frequency. Reports on confusion, delusions, suspicions and hallucinations were recorded from information obtained from the best informed collateral, including relatives, friends, landlords, and physicians; the other items were recorded from the best available source, either the patient or the best informed collateral. Confusion was reported for approximately three-quarters of both men and women, and for both sexes there was an increase in these reports with age. Half the sample refused to eat, drink or take medicine and tended (increasing with age) to have delusions, to be disturbed at night, and to be suspicious. Somewhat more of the younger women (under eighty) than younger men were reported as having delusions and somewhat more of the older women (seventy and over) than men were viewed as being suspicious. Hallucinations, tendencies to get lost or to undertake hazardous activities were recorded for a third of the sample, with no notable sex differences, although the two latter symptoms did increase with age. Symptoms reported for one-tenth to one-third of the sample included tendencies to threaten others, to threaten or to attempt suicide, violence, destructive behaviour, and sexual aberrations. Men were more likely than women to report (or have reported for them) that they threatened others, but this difference is accounted for almost entirely by the youngest men. There are also some age and sex differences for all remaining items in this group: suicide threats tended to decrease with age for both men and women while suicide attempts were reported twice as often by females age sixty to sixty-nine as by males and twice as often by males age seventy to seventy-nine as by females in this age group. Violence toward others was reported twice as frequently for the youngest males as for females, and sexual aberrations were reported four times more often for oldest females than males. Reports of destructive behavior decreased somewhat for both the oldest males and females. In general, disturbances of cognition were reported more often than were behavioral abnormalities. While reports of the former tended to increase with age, reports of the latter tended to decrease with age, particularly in the eighty-and-over age group. Since reports of cognitive disturbances were collected mainly from the best informed collateral, it appears that these disturbances were crucial in contributing to the social definition of mental illness.

We were well aware that yes or no answers to these questions gave us little idea of the intensity with which the symptoms appear and less idea of how they might be interacting with other aspects of the personality. We did learn that, in lieu of any measures of intensity, the mere weight of the number of reported symptoms affords a rough estimate of degree. Nearly one-third of the hospitalized subjects experienced (or were reported to have experienced) six or more symptoms ordinarily considered by clinicians to indicate psychopathology. About one-fourth experienced four or five, and only 18 per cent experienced one. No age trends were apparent for either sex, nor were there any differences between men and women at any age level, except that women tended to have a few more symptoms.

Intellectual functioning. Intellectual status was measured by using both the Kent Emergency Intelligence Test (Kent E-G-Y) (Kent, 1946) and four subtests of the Wechsler Adult Intelligence Scale (WAIS), covering information, comprehension, arithmetic, and digit span (Wechsler, 1955). However, because of the complexity of analyzing test results for a mentally ill sample at time of crisis, data from these tests are not included here. The interested reader is referred to detailed reports by Katz, Neal, and Simon (1961), Crook and Katz (1962), Katz and Crook (1962), Pierce (1963), Trier (1966), Fisher and Pierce (1967a, 1967b). Instead, we report a test of orientation to time, place, and person that was administered by the social interviewers, as one indicator of psychiatric status at time of admission. Before using orientation to measure intellectual status for this book, we did compare it to the Kent E-G-Y and also compared both of these intelligence measures to selected variables in the other four domains and to the outcome. The orientation measure and the Kent E-G-Y were related to each other at less than the .001 level of significance and were associated at the .50 level.[3] Orientation related to our selected variables as well as, and, in most instances, better than the Kent. In general, orientation was more predictive of the patient's status at time of admission to the psychiatric screening wards but the Kent E-G-Y was more predictive of outcome.

The orientation test was administered to 92 per cent of the hospitalized sample, of whom 15 per cent were rated as inaccessible. A patient was considered inaccessible only if he gave no understandable verbal or written response; if he gave an apparently meaningless or garbled response, the words of which could be understood, the answer was recorded. Of the 491 persons tested, 25 per cent were oriented to time, place, and person, 17 per cent were oriented in only two spheres, 39 per cent in only one, and 4 per cent in none. Sex differences occurred only among those oriented in one or none of the spheres: one-half of the females compared to slightly more than one-third of the males. Age and orientation in all three spheres were inversely correlated, whereas age and orientation in only one

[3] The measure of association used here is based on the chi-square statistic as it was introduced by Cramer. It is designated as v by Blalock (1960, p. 230). The advantage of v over the contingency coefficient is that the range of association is always from 0 (independence) to 1 (complete association) regardless of the number of rows and columns. This factor seems particularly important here, where we are comparing variables with varying degrees of freedom.

or in none of the spheres were directly correlated. However, the increases with age for women oriented in only one or no sphere were greater than the proportionate increases for men. The proportion of persons rated inaccessible to testing also increased with age, a relationship which held for both sexes. The oldest men were four times as likely to have been rated inaccessible as the youngest men; the oldest women were only somewhat more likely to have been rated inaccessible than were the youngest women.

PHYSICAL CONDITION

In explaining why the patients were brought to the psychiatric wards, their collateral informants mentioned physical as well as psychiatric problems in three-fourths of all cases. The lay appraisals were confirmed by project psychiatrists. Over two-fifths (42 per cent) were rated as severely impaired, which is defined as "total invalidism for physical reasons or total disability to the degree that the patient requires some form of twenty-four-hour care or supervision." Another two-fifths (41 per cent) were considered moderately impaired, which is defined as having an illness or disability that "definitely limits the patient's capacity to function in some area of everyday living to the degree that he requires some form of assistance or supervision short of twenty-four-hour care." Only 17 per cent were considered mildly impaired. Although their physical impairment might not be as great as their psychiatric impairment, it is obvious that most elderly patients who require emergency psychiatric care in a given year are seriously in need of physical treatment as well. Patients in their sixties and seventies were at least as severely impaired physically as those in their eighties. Partly because of their somewhat lower socioeconomic status, the men were more likely than the women to be severely impaired physically and, conversely, less likely to be only mildly impaired. Sex differences were particularly apparent in the youngest and oldest groups. The somewhat greater physical impairment of the oldest males no doubt results from the greater frequency of chronic brain syndrome associated with arteriosclerotic brain disease; among the very elderly women, chronic brain syndrome is more often associated with senility, a condition which is not necessarily related to physical disorder elsewhere in the soma. The greater frequency of acute brain syndrome among males—a disorder often associated with physical neglect, for example, malnutrition, alcoholism, or untreated congestive heart failure—may account, partly, for discrepancies in the youngest group. While men in the middle age group (seventy to seventy-nine) were less likely to be rated as severely impaired than either the younger or the older men, women in their seventies—in our sample a distinctive group—were more severely impaired than the youngest or oldest of their sex; fully 45 per cent of them were rated severely impaired, while only a third of the youngest and oldest were so rated.

Physical and psychiatric improvement rates during the stay on the screening wards closely resembled each other, and the patients who improved physically were the most likely to improve psychiatrically. Predictably, the patients who improved physically were most likely to be those who had been admitted for alcoholism, acute brain syndrome, or both, and some were recovering from a suicide attempt with overdoses of drugs. Age differences were more related to change in physical condition than were sex differences. Younger men and women were more likely than the older to improve physically while on the ward. Proportionately more of the males who improved were in the sixty to sixty-nine age group whereas proportionately more females who improved were age seventy to seventy-nine. Conversely, the oldest males and females were slightly more likely than the youngest to have remained the same or to have deteriorated physically with few more of the oldest males than females deteriorating. Sixty-three per cent of the patients had been hospitalized for physical reasons during the ten years prior to admission, and, when compared to the community-resident subsample which was matched for age, sex, and socioeconomic status, more than twice as many patients in the hospital subsample reported three or more hospitalizations during the past ten years.

More than 25 per cent of the patients had heart disease and the same number showed signs of marked malnutrition, with which, for more than 33 per cent, went a diagnosis of alcoholism. Thirteen per cent had hypertension and 10 per cent had suffered one or more strokes. Of the 11 per cent who had hearing afflictions, only three-fourths had hearing aids. One-fifth had visual difficulties: nine were blind and the others were suffering from cataracts that lenses could

Table 5
PHYSICAL STATUS INDICATORS BY AGE AND SEX

Physical Domain	Men			Women			Total	
	60–69 %	70–79 %	80+ %	60–69 %	70–79 %	80+ %	Men %	Women %
Impairment								
Mild	15	13	5	30	20	16	13	21
Moderate	38	43	43	38	35	49	41	40
Severe	47	44	52	32	45	35	46	39
N	(75)	(84)	(37)	(58)	(95)	(80)	(196)	(233)
Change on ward								
Improved	21	14	5	16	22	7	15	15
Unchanged	72	75	84	79	71	85	76	78
Deteriorated	7	11	11	5	7	8	9	7
N	(75)	(84)	(37)	(58)	(95)	(80)	(196)	(233)
Diagnoses								
None	17	13	9	28	20	11	14	19
1	37	44	48	37	36	28	42	34
2	25	28	19	20	20	32	25	24
3 or more	21	15	24	15	24	29	19	23
N	(94)	(107)	(46)	(74)	(107)	(97)	(247)	(278)
Reported complaints								
None or 1	19	30	24	24	20	30	24	25
2 or 3	29	34	28	42	31	27	31	32
4 or 5	31	20	26	15	26	26	26	23
6 or more	21	16	22	19	23	17	19	20
N	(96)	(104)	(46)	(74)	(108)	(93)	(246)	(275)

not correct. More women than men, at all age levels, had defective eyesight. Except for those in the very oldest group, men had significantly more respiratory infections; women had significantly more diabetes and fractures. Proportionately more of the youngest men than of the youngest women had peripheral neuritis and cirrhosis of the liver, both of which were associated with alcoholism; the youngest men were also more than twice as likely as the youngest women to suffer from malnutrition. In total number of physical illnesses, there were slight increases in age for females who had three or more.

Patients or their collaterals were asked about various physical symptoms experienced during the year prior to hospitalization, and although these were not as numerous as psychiatric symptoms, only ten per cent had had none at all and 44 per cent had had four or more. Problems reported by one-fourth to one-half of the sample were, in order of frequency: falls or other accidental injuries, weakness or swelling of legs or feet, bowel difficulties (usually constipation), rheumatism or arthritis, fainting spells, headaches, and high blood pressure. Thus, in addition to many specific and serious illnesses, the majority were suffering from a wide array of the more chronic physical insults of aging. Women were more likely than men to suffer from bowel difficulties and rheumatic or arthritic symptoms. And, even though the youngest women were in their sixties, 13 per cent—most within this age group—reported gynecological problems. Men were more likely to have suffered strokes, kidney and bladder (often prostate) problems, and fainting or black-outs, usually in association with alcoholism. Only stroke and kidney or bladder complaints showed a tendency to increase with age. Neither high blood pressure nor rheumatic or arthritic problems showed a tendency to increase with age, perhaps because persons with high blood pressure or rheumatic ailments may die sooner, and thus differences between younger and older groups would be obliterated.

CAPACITY FOR SELF-CARE

Lowenthal (1964a) noted that, for the group of hospitalized persons, problems of management and care played a dominant role in the decisions to admit the patients to the psychiatric wards. Also, one of the major discoveries to arise from the community study

(Lowenthal et al., 1967) was that the community-resident aged who were psychiatrically impaired differed from the hospitalized not so much in the nature of their illnesses or in the amount or nature of the social supports available to them, as in their respective capacities for taking care of their most personal needs themselves, in being able to dress themselves, select their own clothes, take full responsibility for their own health, manage their own money, in general, to be self-sustaining. Immediately before their admission to the screening wards, more than half of the patients needed assistance in moving about on more than one level, in grooming or dressing, in handling money, or in taking care of their own health needs, such as special diets, visits to the doctor, and so on. They also needed supervision for their safety, for example, someone to help them cross streets or to make sure stove burners were turned off. Two-fifths or more needed help in eating, going to the toilet, and bathing. As for a capacity for social interaction, more than half could not respond to verbal overtures by others, and more than two-fifths could only barely use sentences to make themselves understood. Nearly a third were incapable of any kind of response by word or gesture to simple questions.[4]

There is no consistent tendency for the capacity for self-maintenance to decrease with advancing age. As Clark and Anderson (1967) noted in an analysis of the personal and social systems of the mentally ill and the mentally well aged, the presence of mental illness, in this instance often accompanied by physical impairment, tends to obliterate age differences that might be expected in a healthier sample. There were, however, age trends when sex was taken into account. Proportionately more men in their eighties needed toilet assistance than those in their sixties or seventies, but among women those in the seventies rather than the younger or older required assistance. Women in their seventies were also less able to respond to verbal overtures, and there is a definite trend for women in this age group to be less able to care for themselves than either the youngest or oldest women. Men in their sixties and eight-

---

[4] In Chapter Seven is a dichotomy of self-maintenance items which may be heuristically useful: essential functions are bathing, feeding, going to the toilet, health supervision, and safety level; less essential functions are dressing, grooming, locomotion, money management, and household activity.

Table 6

Indicators of Low Self-Maintenance by Age and Sex

Measures of Self-Maintenance	Men			Women			Total	
	60–69 %	70–79 %	80+ %	60–69 %	70–79 %	80+ %	Men %	Women %
Money management (does not handle money)	62	59	71	53	70	68	62	65
N	(86)	(96)	(41)	(68)	(104)	(91)	(223)	(263)
Grooming (partial care of skin, hair, nails)	64	54	61	48	63	63	59	59
N	(83)	(94)	(38)	(69)	(101)	(88)	(215)	(258)
Quality of social activity (unresponsive to social overtures)	56	52	57	43	68	50	54	55
N	(82)	(93)	(40)	(68)	(104)	(90)	(215)	(262)
Dressing (dresses for house only)	52	47	62	41	66	53	52	55
N	(82)	(94)	(40)	(70)	(101)	(89)	(216)	(260)
Safety I (needs hourly supervision)	52	65	55	43	48	48	58	47
N	(81)	(93)	(38)	(65)	(100)	(87)	(212)	(252)

Health (does not care for own health)	53	58	46	46	56	43	52	49
N	(87)	(97)	(39)	(70)	(102)	(91)	(223)	(263)
Locomotion (cannot manage stairs)	48	46	55	40	54	53	49	50
N	(84)	(100)	(42)	(70)	(104)	(93)	(226)	(267)
Expression (does not relate experiences)	39	52	56	38	50	40	48	43
N	(85)	(98)	(41)	(72)	(105)	(93)	(224)	(270)
Bathing (does not wash self)	48	48	39	35	49	36	46	41
N	(82)	(88)	(38)	(66)	(97)	(85)	(208)	(248)
Toilet (needs assistance)	35	37	58	31	53	48	40	45
N	(77)	(88)	(36)	(65)	(94)	(84)	(201)	(243)
Feeding (needs assistance)	36	42	57	31	42	41	42	39
N	(87)	(98)	(40)	(72)	(104)	(93)	(225)	(269)
Safety II (needs supervision in same room)	43	46	41	20	31	30	44	28
N	(84)	(95)	(37)	(70)	(103)	(86)	(216)	(259)
Response (does not respond to questions)	29	31	26	23	39	28	29	31
N	(87)	(99)	(42)	(70)	(101)	(93)	(228)	(264)

ies required more supervision than women in the same age groups and women in their seventies required more care than men in their seventies. Repeatedly in our sample we saw the seventies as a crucial decade for women, with respect to physical and psychiatric deterioration. We have already noted that women in their seventies show similarly higher ratings and more numerous symptoms of both physical and psychiatric disability. To some extent, differences in the nature of their psychiatric illnesses may account for the greater impairment of women who are in their seventies. Psychogenic disorder, with or without organic brain syndrome, is similar in men and women who are in their sixties or eighties. In their seventies, women are considerably more likely than men to suffer from organic brain syndrome without accompanying psychogenic disorder (70 per cent, compared with 54 per cent). Why such diagnostic differences occur is puzzling.

PSYCHOSOCIAL CHARACTERISTICS

Of the many questions bearing on psychosocial characteristics, we selected primarily those designed to test certain hypotheses about the importance of age-linked stresses, and those that, in the community study (Lowenthal et al., 1967), distinguished most strongly between the mentally ill and the mentally well. As a whole, the screening ward sample did not differ notably from elderly San Franciscans in general in the few characteristics on which census data are available.

More of the hospitalized group than of all San Franciscans sixty or older were widowed largely because of their advanced age. When we compared them with a community-resident subsample matched for age, sex, and socioeconomic status, there were no differences, thus shedding doubt on the validity of our hypothesis that the age-linked stress of widowhood may trigger mental illness for which hospitalization is necessary. This hypothesis was further shaken by the fact that three-fifths of the hospitalized widowed group, who amounted to 39 per cent of the total sample, but consisted of almost three times as many widows as widowers, had been widowed for twenty or more years prior to their admission to the screening wards. Only 5 per cent had been widowed for less than five years. Nor was this one of the sociopsychological stresses contributing to the more marked disabilities of the women in the middle age group: 40 per cent of the widows were in their seventies and, of those, only 6 per cent had been widowed for fewer than ten years (none fewer than five) and nearly two-thirds had been widowed for twenty or more years. There were even more widows among women in their eighties, and they were less debilitated than were the younger women. Men were somewhat more likely to have been rather recently widowed—8 per cent within five years prior to admission, compared with 3 per cent among the women. Thus, if the hypothesis has any validity, it would appear that widowhood may be a triggering or predisposing stress for men more often than it is for women, though as Lowenthal showed (1964b), it is not likely to be reported as such.

The other age-linked social stress is retirement. All but a handful of the patients were retired, even those under sixty-five (of whom only 15 per cent had been working within a year of hospitalization). An examination of the raw data suggested that retirement might be somewhat more related to the onset of mental illness in old age than is widowhood: more than 33 per cent of the men and women who had worked for twenty years or more had retired within five years of admission, 15 per cent within two years. However, a chronological analysis (Lowenthal, 1965) of the course of the illness in relation to the timing of various other changes in the patients' lives indicated that, by and large, among those suffering from psychogenic as well as among those suffering from organic brain disorder, retirement took place after the first symptoms of the illness began to develop.

There were no very dramatic differences between men and women or in the three age groups in actual or potential social supports available to them prior to admission, except that men tended to be more deprived than women on the scale of socioeconomic status at all age levels, and to report their current living standard as much worse than at age fifty. The women—despite their higher socioeconomic status—tended to have had less education than the men. Sex differences were especially noticeable among those in their eighties: far more than half of the men had had at least some high school education compared with only a fourth of the women. There were no differences between men and women in their sixties.

Women in their seventies tended to be at the extremes: there were more with a higher education (some high school or more) and more with a lower education (less than eighth grade) than those in their sixties or eighties.

There were no marked age or sex differences in regard to having children, though men were more likely to live at some distance from their children than were women. No doubt partly because they were more likely to be married, men tended to have more social roles than women, and for them the number of such roles did not decline with age. Forty-seven per cent of the women in their sixties had two or more social roles, whereas only 24 per cent of those in their eighties had that many. (Roles include those of spouse, parent, church member, worker, organization member.) Although more men were married, a few more men than women lived alone prior to admission (48 per cent, compared with 44 per cent). The women, however, because of their more advanced age and the greater frequency of senility among them, were slightly more likely to have been in institutions such as nursing homes prior to admission to the screening wards than were men (17 per cent, compared with 13 per cent). Nearly half of the group (48 per cent) had had contact with a community social agency, but mainly for monetary reasons only, for example, public welfare. Among women, such contacts increased with age, from one-third of the sixty-year-olds to more than half of those in their eighties. Among men, age differences were negligible.

Men were more likely to be foreign-born than were women, and of the men seventy or older, more than half were foreign-born, compared with about two-fifths of the women. This tendency was reversed in the youngest group, age sixty to sixty-nine: only 29 per cent of the men, compared with 38 per cent of the women, were foreign-born. This discrepancy may in part be explained by the fact that native-born males are more likely to become alcoholic than are foreign-born males and most of the alcoholics in the sample were found among the younger males.

In keeping with findings from other studies (Z. Blau, 1961), women maintained more social contacts than men, more than half of them (56 per cent) having visited or been visited by friends or relatives in the two weeks before admission, compared with only 40 per cent of the men. These differences held for all three age groups, but were less dramatic among people in their eighties. The women in their seventies, who were more impaired on several counts than the younger or older women, and than men in their seventies, were socially more active than other women and than all men.

Religious differences between the hospitalized sample and the elderly in the community at large were not notable, except that persons of the Jewish faith were somewhat under-represented. However, there was a tendency, difficult to explain, for the proportion of Catholics to increase with advancing age. This was particularly noticeable among men—where 34 per cent of those in their sixties, compared with 51 per cent of those in their eighties, reported that they were Catholics. Women in their seventies were somewhat different; they were rather more likely to be Protestant or Jewish than were the younger or older women or than were the men in their own age group.

Two subjective characteristics that tended to distinguish rather markedly between the mentally ill and the mentally well among the community-resident aged (Lowenthal et al., 1967) were those of self-concept and of the tendency to complain about various inconveniences in living arrangements. Questions about self-concept were asked only at the time of the first follow-up interview, so discussion of it will be deferred. Inconveniences or potential inconveniences that were noted included: no room of one's own; no control of heat regulation; the sharing of a toilet and/or a bath and their being on a different floor from the bedroom, or in a different dwelling unit; steps within the dwelling unit or between it and the street; living alone. The tendency in the community sample to complain about such arrangements was found to vary quite dramatically between the ill and the well even when the number of such inconveniences was held constant.

Such questions could be asked only of persons who were responsive and could function fairly well intellectually—less than half of the sample. Perhaps for this reason proneness to complain, which proved to be an important characteristic in the deprivation index that discriminated between the mentally ill and the mentally well in the community, proved less useful for the hospitalized mentally ill. Although the hospitalized in fact suffered more of these potential inconveniences, only 20 per cent of those able to respond complained about them, compared with nearly one-third of the community sample. Among the community-resident aged, furthermore, those who complained were twice as likely to be mentally impaired as those who did not, which suggested that proneness to stress may be a significant factor in the development of mental illness. Two special conditions of the hospitalized patients may be involved in their apparent satisfacton with their living arrangements. First, the primary objective of the elderly patients who were fairly intact mentally while they were on the screening wards was to return to their community residence rather than to go to a state hospital. To admit of any problems would have been to cast doubt on the adequacy of their homes. Second, their psychiatric and physical problems were so severe that matters such as inconveniences in their living arrangements may well have paled in comparison. A few trends, however, are notable. Women tended to complain more than men (24 per cent, compared with 16 per cent who referred to one or more inconveniences). The men's tendency to make such complaints decreased with age; only half as many men in their eighties made such complaints as men in their sixties. However, more women in their eighties complained than did women in their sixties; the peak was reached by women in their seventies, who proved to be the most complaint-prone of any age and sex group, and twice as much so as men in their seventies.

SUMMARY

Elderly patients who undergo psychiatric crises for the first time after age sixty suffer for the most part from massive disintegration, generally physical as well as psychiatric. The assistance that would have been needed to maintain them as "going concerns," to borrow Williams' phrase (1961, p. 268) was considerable. All needed assistance in at least one vital area of self-maintenance, and most in several. Regardless of the nature of their illness, intellectually they were performing at a considerably lower level than is considered normal for their age.

We found no convincing evidence for the hypothesis that age-linked stresses such as widowhood or retirement trigger illnesses or hospitalizations in old age, but there was some evidence, from our examination of six age- and sex-groups, that different cohorts are involved. The most striking deviations from the sample as a whole were found among the youngest men and among the women in their seventies. The former were characterized by lower socio-economic status, a higher proportion of the native-born and of Protestants, and by certain signs of social isolation such as living alone, low social interaction, and a higher proportion of separation or divorce—all characteristics that fit the classic pattern of the Skid Row alcoholic, which, in fact, many of the men were. The women in the middle range (age seventy to seventy-nine), however, deviated even more strikingly: they were more seriously impaired on many counts than were either the younger or the older women and than men in their own age group. They tended to have either less or more education, to include more Jews and Protestants, and to be more complaint-prone. At the same time, they maintained a higher level of social interaction than any other age- and sex-group. They were more likely than men of the same age to be suffering from organic brain syndrome without accompanying psychogenic disorder. Among men, the principal psychogenic disorder was alcoholism, but since it is unlikely that lack of alcoholism can account for the more severe impairment of women, one is tempted to speculate about the significance, first, of the women's higher degree of social interaction and, second, of their complaint- or stress-proneness. It may be that these women in their seventies were or had been more achievement-oriented than other age- and sex-groups. More of them worked than did younger and older women, and despite more severe impairment, more of them maintained a fairly high degree of social interaction just prior to admission. Some of them may well have been striving over-achievers, and possibly were less flexible, and less tolerant of the aging process. If they were particularly stress-prone, as their responses to the complaint question suggested, it may be also that history had left its mark on them, for these women who, in their seventies in 1959, were at crucial ages during the major cataclysms of this century: during World War I, their husbands might have been drafted, leaving them with very young children; during the Depression, demands for the children's education might have been greatest (they were also in the menopausal period at that time); during World War II, many of them had sons of draft age, and, among the small group of Jews, some were uprooted from their home countries late in life. Finally, born in the 1880's, they were perhaps at a particularly impressionable age at the peak of the Feminist Movement which encouraged women to assert their independence.

CHAPTER THREE

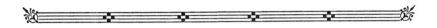

Clinical Diagnoses

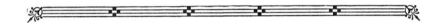

Diagnosis is discussed in this chapter to give greater clarity to the various formal clinical categories; to give more detail about the two major categories (psychogenic and organic disorders) used in the rest of the book; to show the bases on which the clinical diagnoses were made and how patients were placed in one or another category when the history was meager or unobtainable and the patient unable to provide the necessary information; to indicate the close correlation between clinical diagnosis and prognosis and the usefulness of a multi-diagnostic formulation; to indicate the frequency and importance of physical illness in mentally ill elderly patients who are admitted to hospitals; and to emphasize the frequency of alcoholism among the geriatric mentally ill.

When the initial data were gathered, in 1959, the official psychiatric nomenclature in use was the 1952 *Diagnostic and Statistical Manual* of the American Psychiatric Association (DMS-1). Table 7 shows the relationship of the diagnostic categories used by our project, those of DMS-1, and those in the 1968 revised edition

Table 7

DIAGNOSTIC CATEGORIES

Geriatric Research Project	Diagnostic and Statistical Manual	
	1952	1968
Organic Brain Syndromes	*Organic Brain Syndromes*	*Organic Brain Syndromes*
Acute Brain Syndromes	Acute Brain Syndromes	Acute Brain Syndromes
Chronic Brain Syndromes	Chronic Brain Syndromes	Chronic Brain Syndromes
Psychogenic Disorders	*Psychoneurotic Disorders*	*Neuroses*
Depressive Disorders	Depressive Reaction	Depressive Neurosis
	Psychotic Disorders	*Psychoses not attributed to physical conditions listed previously*
	Involutional Psychotic Reaction	
	Affective Reactions	*Major Affective Disorders*
	Manic Depressive Reaction (depressed type)	Manic Depressive Illness

		Involutional Melancholia
Paranoid Disorders	Psychotic Depressive Reaction	Psychotic Depressive Reaction
	Schizophrenic Reactions (paranoid type)	Schizophrenia (paranoid type)
	Paranoid Reactions	Paranoid States Involutional Paranoid State
	Paranoia Paranoid State	Paranoia Other Paranoid States
Personality Disorders	*Personality Disorders*	*Personality Disorders and certain other non-psychotic Mental Disorders*
Personality Pattern Disorders	Personality Pattern Disturbances Personality Trait Disturbances	Personality Disorders
Alcoholism	Sociopathic Personality Alcoholism	Alcoholism
Transient Situational Reactions	Transient Situational Personality Disorders	Transient Situational Disturbances

(DMS-2). The similarities between the project diagnostic categories and those in the two diagnostic manuals are obvious; the major difference is the grouping of depressive and paranoid diagnoses into two large categories rather than into the smaller subtypes specified in the manuals.

Throughout most of this book, the diagnostic categories used are psychogenic disorder and organic brain disorder. Primary diagnosis is mentioned where the interest is in the disorder that actually led to hospitalization, regardless of any additional diagnoses or of the duration or severity of any other disorders present. Table 8 gives diagnostic breakdown of the sample that indicates the major clinical categories found. Here the alcoholics are placed in a separate cate-

Table 8

DIAGNOSTIC GROUPS: HOSPITAL SAMPLE

	Number	*Percentage*
Acute Brain Syndrome, no Chronic Brain Syndrome (no alcoholics)	29	5
Chronic Brain Syndrome, no Acute Brain Syndrome (no alcoholics)	155	29
Acute Brain Syndrome plus Chronic Brain Syndrome (no alcoholics)	173	32
Alcoholics	122	23
Psychogenic Disorder Only	46	9
Undiagnosed	9	2
Total	(534)	100

gory, partly to emphasize the frequency and importance of alcoholism among the geriatric mentally ill and partly because, even when organic brain syndromes were diagnosed, if alcoholism were a prominent part of the clinical picture, the course of illness followed a pattern more closely resembling that characteristic of psychogenic disorders than that of senile or arteriosclerotic brain syndromes. The alcoholics are drawn from almost all the other diagnostic categories but, even though they constituted a much larger percentage of the psychogenics, the basic differences between the psychogenic and the organic groups could not be attributed to the alcoholics, nor, for that matter, to age (Trier, 1966).

As many as three psychiatric diagnoses were given to each patient, together with diagnoses of physical illnesses serious enough to interfere with functioning. Multiple diagnosis provided a clearer clinical picture of each patient, and proved to have prognostic significance. The primary diagnosis was that of the condition that, in the judgment of the examining psychiatrist, precipitated the patient's admission to the screening ward. Secondary and tertiary diagnoses were made in the order of relative importance to the overall clinical condition of the patient. The major precipitating condition was acute brain syndrome (53 per cent of the sample); next was chronic brain syndrome (27 per cent), followed by psychogenic disorder (20 per cent). If the alcoholics were disregarded entirely, acute brain syndrome would account for only 37 per cent of the admissions. However, because five-sixths of the 122 alcoholics had acute brain syndromes, the figure was raised to 53 per cent.

ACUTE BRAIN SYNDROME

The following definition of acute brain syndrome was used by project psychiatrists when assigning diagnoses to patients in the sample: "Usually of abrupt onset, seldom lasting more than one month before admission. Characterized by: fluctuating disturbances in consciousness, varying from mild confusion to stupor and coma; impairment of intellectual functioning, principally memory disturbance and disorientation; in some cases delusions, illusions, and hallucinations; pathologic emotional states such as fear, apprehension, emotional lability, irritability, or apathy; physiologic disturbance, the onset of which was associated with the psychiatric upset. The symptom complex may be completely reversible if the underlying physiologic disturbance can be corrected, or it may indicate a terminal state, as in cardiac failure, uremia, certain malignancies, or the sequelae of a cerebrovascular accident. It may be superimposed on a long-term chronic brain syndrome that is revealed if the manifestations of the acute brain syndrome clear. The latter group includes patients with only brief, transient episodes of noisy, restless, and disturbed behavior during a senile or arteriosclerotic psychosis if the episodes are associated with a physiologic disturbance such as cardiac failure or cerebrovascular accident."

This unusually broad diagnostic category of acute brain syndrome subsumes many of the acute physiologic disturbances that sometimes are thought to be part of the symptomatic course of geriatric mental illnesses associated with chronic structural and physiologic changes in the brain. Because of their underlying mental illness, patients with chronic brain syndromes often tend to neglect their health, seldom seek medical attention, may suffer from malnutrition and vitamin deficiency, and are, therefore, more susceptible to acute physiologic disturbances that may precipitate a transient acute brain syndrome.

The physiologic disturbances most commonly associated with acute brain syndromes $(N = 288)$ in this sample were: malnutrition $(N = 85)$, cardiac failure $(N = 61)$, alcohol $(N = 44)$, cerebrovascular accident $(N = 29)$, drugs and toxins $(N = 12)$, trauma $(N = 4)$, uremia $(N = 4)$, surgery $(N = 2)$, pulmonary disease $(N = 2)$, cancer $(N = 2)$, and conditions such as convulsive disorder, hypertensive arteriosclerosis, diffuse collagen disease, and so forth $(N = 43)$. These illnesses were serious enough to interfere with the patients' function and were closely associated with the clinical and behavioral symptoms that were interpreted as indicating acute brain syndrome. As well as the patients whose physical illnesses were associated with acute brain syndromes, there were many with similar illnesses of less severity and not associated with the clinical psychiatric symptomatology. In all, four-fifths of the sample of 534 were found to be suffering from moderate or severe physical disability as a result of physical illness.

> *Case.*   Mr. Gray, age sixty-four, was married at the time of admission and living with his third wife. He had been a salesman and for fifteen years before his retirement had worked at a variety of low-paying jobs. He suffered from "heart trouble" for several years prior to admission. Six years before admission a subtotal gastrectomy was performed because of a peptic ulcer. He had overindulged in alcohol intermittently for many years. For several days before admission he had appeared "dazed," had become "nervous and restless," was more irritable, and tended to ramble in his conversation. A physician

recommended admission to a hospital for "heart treatment." On the medical ward of the general hospital, Mr. Gray suddenly developed a "delirious episode." A recent myocardial infarction was diagnosed. The patient was reported to have said that a "mad Russian with a beard" was at his bedside "trying to kill" him. He described auditory and visual hallucinations and was confused and disoriented. He was transferred to the psychiatric screening ward, but within two days, his psychiatric symptoms cleared. His diagnosis was acute brain syndrome associated with cardiac decompensation and a recent myocardial infarction. (638)*

When acute brain syndrome was superimposed on a chronic brain syndrome, the acute brain syndrome differed in duration prior to admission from cases in which there was acute brain syndrome only. The acute brain syndrome averaged twice as long prior to admission in patients with combined acute and chronic brain syndromes (15.25 days) as in patients with only acute brain syndrome (6.25 days). Most cases of long duration were attributed to malnutrition, a few to alcohol. Apparently, if a geriatric patient's disturbance becomes severe only gradually, it is more easily tolerated than is a sudden behavioral disturbance which is more likely to make his caretakers anxious. Although it is our impression that repeated episodes of physiologic decompensation tended to speed up the deteriorative process, the data available were not sufficient to establish this firmly. As an acute brain syndrome is associated with a serious physiologic disturbance, there is a high mortality during the first month following hospitalization among patients with acute brain syndrome only and patients with an associated chronic brain syndrome.

Because the behavioral symptoms associated with acute brain syndrome often are the presenting feature that brings the patient to the hospital or to the attention of a physician, the accompanying physical illness may be overlooked or minimized and the symptoms interpreted as evidence of chronic brain syndrome rather than of acute physiologic decompensation. Disturbed behavior in such patients is a function not only of the underlying physical illness or of chronic brain syndrome but also of the patient's personality and

* Numbers in parentheses at the end of case studies are case numbers.

of his reaction to impaired cerebral function and to the interpersonal situation in which he lives.

> *Case.* Mrs. Crane, age seventy-three, had been widowed for fifteen years. She lived alone in a house, went to church every day, rarely talked to or visited with others, and had her principal contacts with her daughter and her family. The daughter took her meals to her daily and saw "that she was properly taken care of." In the year prior to admission, she seemed to be getting gradually weaker and became unable to care for herself. Two weeks before admission, she suddenly declared that someone was trying to kill her. She thought she heard voices calling her bad names. The daughter reported that the patient "wanted to go to Heaven—she heard angels talking to her all night—she was afraid I would poison her—she did not know me—she could not remember anything—her memory had been getting worse in the last year, and she accused a woman friend of being a man and trying to rape her." On admission, Mrs. Crane appeared confused and disoriented, her memory was markedly impaired, she was irritable and at times angry. She verbalized paranoid, hallucinatory, and delusional ideas. Physical examination and laboratory tests revealed hypertension, generalized arteriosclerosis, and pyelonephritis. Her diagnosis was chronic brain syndrome, senile type, with superimposed acute brain syndrome associated with pyelonephritis. (632)

Alcoholism. A diagnosis of acute brain syndrome associated with alcoholism was made when the classical signs of acute brain syndrome were apparent and were associated with a history of recent heavy drinking. A diagnosis of chronic brain syndrome associated with alcoholism was made when the history indicated heavy drinking, usually of several years' duration, and gradual social and intellectual deterioration of months' to years' duration. Notwithstanding such a history, if focal neurologic signs secondary to stroke were present, diagnostic preference was given to cerebral arteriosclerosis as the cause of the chronic brain syndrome. When the patient was more than seventy years old and had no history or evidence of focal neurologic damage, diagnostic preference was likely to be given to senile brain disease, regardless of the alcoholic history. Admittedly, this differential diagnosis is difficult, and its accuracy can be established finally only by detailed postmortem examination.

Although in the general population the proportion of alcoholics decreases with advancing age (Knupfer and Room, 1964), more elderly alcoholics are admitted to the psychiatric wards of a general hospital than is generally realized (Simon, Epstein, and Reynolds, 1968). The 122 alcoholics in the sample (23 per cent) fell into three large groups evidenced by: alcoholism, with no chronic brain syndrome and almost universal acute brain syndrome (42 per cent of the alcoholics); alcoholism with alcoholic chronic brain syndrome (38 per cent of the alcoholics); and alcoholism with senile or arteriosclerotic chronic brain syndrome (20 per cent of the alcoholics). Almost three-fourths of the alcoholics were admitted with acute brain syndromes, nearly all of which were associated with excessive and prolonged drinking. About two-thirds of the alcoholics had associated chronic brain syndromes, most of which were alcoholic brain syndromes. Although the proportion of alcoholics in this sample seems quite large, it is comparable to the 20 per cent found by Whittier and Korenyi (1961) in a sample of 540 male first admissions over the age of sixty in a New York State mental hospital. The problem may be more characteristic of large urban populations than of rural or less urbanized populations. In contrast to patients with senile or arteriosclerotic chronic brain syndromes, the alcoholics tended to be discharged to the community rather than to remain in hospitals.

Suicide. Coroner's records for 1959 showed sixty-three successful suicides in the age group sixty and over. San Francisco General Hospital records showed thirty-one patients admitted because of suicide attempts in 1959, of whom thirteen were in the hospital sample and ten in the group of ineligibles. Fifteen patients in the hospital sample had attempted suicide recorded as at least one reason for admission, and five patients had attempted suicide at some time in the few months prior to admission. Eighty-one patients in the sample had threatened suicide during the few months prior to admission but did not make an actual attempt. The thirteen patients in the sample who were admitted as suicide attempters received admission diagnoses of acute brain syndrome (in all cases the result

of an ingestion of drugs or poisons, mostly barbiturates) and diagnoses of depression. Three patients were diagnosed as having, in
addition, chronic brain syndromes. All the suicidal patients were
admitted in comatose or semi-comatose states that were serious
enough, especially in view of the suicide attempt, to warrant admission to a psychiatric screening ward. The presenting symptoms usually cleared within twenty-four to seventy-two hours, after which
the underlying depressive condition was clearly evident. In the three
cases in which diagnoses of chronic brain syndromes also were
given, the evidence for the chronic brain syndrome was equivocal,
and the condition, if actually present, was mild.

Guns were used extensively by the successful suicides, but
by none of the attempters. The most common methods used by the
successful suicides were barbiturates (29 per cent), gunshot (22
per cent, all men), hanging (17 per cent), and jumping, other than
from the Golden Gate Bridge (14 per cent). Among the attempters,
the most commonly used methods were barbiturates (31 per cent),
other ingestion (29 per cent), razor or knife (13 per cent, almost
all men), and jumping, other than from the Golden Gate Bridge
(11 per cent).

CHRONIC BRAIN SYNDROME

The following definitions of chronic brain syndromes of various types were used by project psychiatrists when assigning diagnoses to patients in the sample: "History of gradual intellectual and
personality disorganization extending from months to several years.
Characterized by: disturbances in comprehension, memory, and orientation; in many cases, emotional instability, irritability, anxiety,
apathy, and hallucinations or delusions."

Senile brain syndrome. Onset after age sixty-five; history
of gradual and progressive inability to deal with day-to-day life.
Associated with clinical evidence of intellectual deterioration of
months' to years' duration; no history or neurologic evidence of one
or more cerebrovascular accidents or evidence of chronic alcoholic,
syphilitic, or other brain disease or post-traumatic conditions.

Case. Mr. Lewis, age seventy-seven, was admitted to the
hospital with symptoms of "disorganized behavior, disorientation, and lack of cooperation." He had lived in San Francisco

all his life and was a retired jewelry salesman. His wife had been hospitalized with a heart attack one week before his admission to the psychiatric screening ward. His son reported that "his mental faculties have been lapsing for the last six or seven years." However, it was not until about a year before admission that Mr. Lewis was discharged from his job because he was making so many mistakes. During the year prior to admission, he needed close and constant supervision, even for such basic functions as eating and dressing properly. Although his wife had been hospitalized, he continued to believe that she was home in the apartment. When interviewed shortly after admission, he insisted that he was not ill, that he was not in a hospital, that he did not know who had brought him there, that he had been here for the last three weeks and—a sentence later—that he had just arrived a short time ago. Almost no factual information could be obtained from him. The son reported that he had not realized how deteriorated his father had become until he found him home alone when his mother had to go to the hospital. There was no history of stroke or fainting spells. This patient was admitted primarily because his wife was no longer at home to care for him and the family could not. The results of physical and neurologic examinations were unremarkable. Laboratory tests were essentially negative. An X-ray of the skull showed a massive enlargement of the sela turcica, and it was suspected that the patient might have a chromophobe adenoma. His diagnosis was chronic brain syndrome, senile type, with psychotic reaction. Mr. Lewis was transferred to a state mental hospital, where he died of terminal bronchial penumonia one year after admission. Neuropathologic studies indicated severe senile brain disease with associated mild arteriosclerotic brain disease and idiopathic calcification of the globus pallidus. There was no evidence of a chromophobe adenoma. (272)

Arteriosclerotic brain syndrome. Intellectual deterioration of months' to years' duration associated with focal neurologic signs and symptoms found in the case history of clinical findings or both, and secondary to one or more cerebrovascular accidents (probably atherosclerotic in origin). Included are patients with histories of fluctuating course, usually early in the illness, or one or more seizures often associated with severe hypertension (probably with cerebral arteriolar changes). A history of headaches and dizziness in the early stages is frequent.

Case. Mrs. Hardy was a seventy-seven-year-old married woman. Her seventy-nine-year-old husband reported that his wife began to have "falls" one and one-half years prior to admission, her blood pressure, which was "up to 250" had caused "dizzy spells and blackouts; her mind had become increasingly impaired," she became more and more confused, especially during the five months before admission, and she seemed to be living in the past. Her health had been good. Because of the repeated falls, she had been admitted, eleven days before, to a nursing home where she became acutely disoriented and disorganized, and was screaming and unmanageable. On admission, she was disoriented, showed evidence of global memory loss, did not know that she was in the hospital, did not remember being in a nursing home, tended to perseverate, and her thinking was markedly slow. A physical examination revealed evidence of generalized arteriosclerosis, hypertension, a right hemiparesis, and bilateral cataracts. Her diagnosis was chronic brain syndrome associated with cerebral arteriosclerosis, with associated generalized arteriosclerosis and hypertension. (534)

Chronic alcoholic brain syndrome. History of excessive alcohol indulgence and nutritional deficiency over many years and evidence of intellectual deterioration (with or without a Korsakoff-like syndrome) of months' to years' duration. Because of the definite history of excessive alcoholism and nutritional deficiency, the intellectual deterioration is attributed to neuropathologic changes secondary to alcoholism rather than to senile brain disease. Such patients are likely to be younger (sixty-five to seventy-five) than patients diagnosed as having senile brain syndromes. Peripheral neuritis may or may not be present.

Case. Mr. Jones, a sixty-nine-year-old divorced man, worked as a mail handler for the post office and retired at the age of sixty after thirty-two years of service. His daughter reported that he drank even while working. He lived a comparatively isolated life, without visits from friends or relatives except for his daughter, who described him as "a violent drunk and not easy to get along with." He was referred to the hospital by the police on the complaint of his daughter, who said, "He has been alcoholic for forty years. A few days ago he began having hallucinations and became confused. He was in DT's for a couple of days, and then he got worse. We could not get the doctor, so we called the police. We were afraid of what he might do. He will kill me or my children or somebody. He was having hallucinations; he saw Jesus Christ and he started to tear the walls down." On the ward, the day after admission, he appeared eager to talk and spoke rapidly but often irrelevantly. He knew that he was in the hospital, but could not name it and was unable to name the current president of the United States. He told a rambling story about Mexicans who came into his room and took his money, and then added that his daughter had shanghaied him to be a witness against a Mexican woman. Physical examination revealed an enlarged liver, marked intention tremor, generalized muscular atrophy, decreased deep tendon reflexes, hyperalgesia and hypethesia over the lower extremities, and moderate ataxia in walking. It was believed that he showed evidence of peripheral neuritis. His diagnosis was acute brain syndrome associated with alcohol, superimposed upon a mild to moderately severe chronic brain syndrome associated with alcoholism. (507)

Other chronic brain syndromes. Other patients with chronic brain syndromes suffered from a number of conditions, of months' to years' duration, including trauma, convulsive disorder, idiopathic Parkinsonism, and central nervous system syphilis. In some cases, the origin of the chronic brain syndrome was undetermined.

Neuropathology. The relationship between structural brain changes and mental deterioration in the aged has been uncertain. Gellerstedt (1933) and Rothschild (1937) both reported a lack of correlation between the intensity of clinical symptoms and the severity of brain disease—an erroneous conclusion: there is a gross but definite correlation. Rothschild may have been misled because cognitive functions are more closely correlated with the degree of neuropathology than is the total clinical picture. Behavior disturbances are not necessarily related to the severity of neuropathologic changes and may or may not be a reaction to cognitive deficit. Corsellis (1962) reported a high correlation between clinical diagnosis and neuropathologic changes, and his findings are supported by Malamud (1942) and Simon and Malamud (1968). Roth and his co-workers (Roth, Tomlinson, and Blessed, 1966) also reported a high correlation between certain quantitative measures of intellectual and personality deterioration in the aged and density of senile plaque formation in the brain.

The mere existence of cerebral arteriosclerosis is not the important feature in its relation to mental symptoms. The essential features are the presence of infarctions, which are usually multiple, and the amount of brain damage. There may be considerable cerebral arteriosclerosis with little or no brain damage. The neuropathology of geriatric mental illness is not limited to senile and arteriosclerotic brain disease. In a study (Simon, 1962) of 505 elderly patients admitted to a state mental hospital who were diagnosed as suffering from senile or cerebral arteriosclerotic psychoses, approximately 11 per cent were determined neuropathologically to have had brain changes associated with such other conditions as Pick's Disease, "toxic" encephalopathy, "chronic Wernicke's" encephalopathy, brain tumor, brain aneurysm, and so forth. Of our 328 patients diagnosed as suffering from chronic organic brain syndromes other than those associated with alcoholism, 49 per cent were diagnosed as having senile brain syndrome only, 32 per cent as having arteriosclerotic brain syndrome only, 13 per cent as having combined senile and arteriosclerotic brain syndromes, and 6 per cent as having chronic brain syndromes of other types. This is remarkably close to the proportions of such conditions found on neuropathologic examination in Simon's study. Simon showed also that, although the psychiatrists in the state mental hospital had diagnosed accurately the presence or absence of organic brain syndrome (in fact, in only 3.5 per cent of the cases was no definite neuropathology found), the specific type of brain syndrome (senile, arteriosclerotic, and so forth) generally was not accurately diagnosed clinically. This could well be true for our sample, even though the proportions turned out to be so close to those in the neuropathologic study.

Differential diagnosis. Diagnosis depends on a detailed and reasonably accurate history from the patient or from collaterals. Such histories were not always available for our sample, even from family members, as a significant number of patients lived alone, sometimes with little or no contact with families. A diagnosis of cerebral arteriosclerosis, in particular, depends on a reasonably accurate history of previous strokes, which do not always leave permanent neurologic signs. In cases where no objective evidence of focal neurologic damage can be found, especially in older patients, the more likely diagnosis was senile brain syndrome. A number of patients suffered from combined senile and arteriosclerotic brain disease. The tendency in such cases was to diagnose senile brain syndrome if the patient were seventy-five years old or older. If a patient in his seventies begins to show evidence of gradual impairment of orientation, memory, and intellectual function and, after several years suffers a cerebrovascular accident, one may assume that a senile process has been going on and has been complicated by cerebral arteriosclerosis that has resulted in a cerebral thrombosis. In such an instance, a diagnosis of combined senile-arteriosclerotic brain syndrome could be made. However, if the onset of the patient's chronic brain syndrome is associated with a stroke, one is much less likely to diagnose senile brain disease, since the symptoms resulting from senile brain disease would be obscured by those resulting from cerebrovascular disease.

Many depressed and paranoid patients do badly on psychologic tests and on the tests commonly used by the physician to evaluate memory, orientation, and intellectual functioning, because of the inhibition imposed by depression or the suspicion, anger, and lack of cooperation associated with paranoid reactions. Thus frequently it is difficult to be certain whether the apparent cognitive impairment is the result of behavioral and emotional components or of underlying neuropathologic processes. With improvement in the behavioral and psychogenic aspects of the illness, the apparent cognitive impairment may improve or disappear. In the presence of affective or paranoid components, the manifestations of impaired intellectual functioning are generally mild, and certainly are no more than moderate. When intellectual impairment is severe, depressive and paranoid symptomatology are rarely present. When psychogenic disorder appears in combination with chronic brain syndrome, the brain syndrome tends to be mild or, at most, moderate. In general, prognosis follows a course determined by the psychogenic disorder rather than by the chronic brain syndrome, especially in relation to mortality and the frequency of placement in the community.

> *Case.* Mr. Murphy, a seventy-year-old married man, began showing signs of a failing memory approximately a year before his hospitalization. Six months before, two of his brothers died, one shortly after the other, and the patient became in-

creasingly depressed and preoccupied with his own health. He became irritable and more withdrawn, and developed fears "of losing his soul." He wanted to go to confession all the time, and worried over his health. His wife stated that he became "very confused, could not remember things, and he thinks I am his sister sometimes." Because his wife suffered from severe arthritis and was unable to care for the patient any longer, he was admitted to the hospital. In the hospital he was uncooperative, constantly demanding to see a priest and refusing to answer many of the inquiries made of him. He was disoriented as to place and time, and apart from his suspicious and belligerent attitude, the examiner was impressed by his inability to recall many events in his past life. He tended to avoid responding to anything that was a problem for him to solve. The results of a physical examination were essentially negative, except for a systolic murmur over the precordium and tremors of the outstretched hand. He was transferred to a state mental hospital, where he was given a course of electroshock therapy and showed improvement in his depressive symptomatology, but continued to be "confused." His intellectual functions deteriorated. Five months after admission he suddenly suffered a right hemiplegia with a complicating pneumonitis and died a few days later. His diagnosis was acute psychotic depressive reaction superimposed on a mild chronic brain syndrome, senile type. The subsequent cerebrovascular accident would indicate an underlying cerebral arteriosclerosis. (521)

PSYCHOGENIC DISORDERS

Psychogenic disorders include those called "functional" or mental disorders not attributed to physical conditions, that is, all conditions not specifically listed as organic brain syndromes.

Affective disorders. Depressive reactions (manic-depressive, involutional, neurotic, reactive, or psychotic), whether or not recurrent. If the depressed patient has attempted suicide by poison or drugs, thus causing an acute brain syndrome, the primary diagnosis is acute brain syndrome, the secondary one depressive reaction. As the differentiation between manic-depressive, involutional, and other types of depression is often artificial, and because only a few patients were diagnosed in each of these categories in our sample, the cases were combined into one group labeled "affective disorders." These patients' symptoms are primarily those of a mood disorder (depression) frequently associated with anxiety; agitation; insomnia (often early morning waking); indecision; subjective complaints of difficulty in concentration, memory, and thinking; feelings of hopelessness; suicidal thoughts; self-derogatory and self-deprecatory feelings; guilt feelings; somatic complaints, especially constipation; and sometimes somatic delusions.

> *Case.* Mrs. Martin was a sixty-four-year-old divorced woman. Her health had been "fair" except for diabetes that she had had for twenty-four years and that had been treated by a combination of insulin and diet or by diet alone. Recently, she had not been using insulin and was not eating properly. During the three months prior to admission she had become increasingly nervous and depressed. She did not want to see or talk to anyone, and she paced up and down in her room because she was "so nervous." She was afraid she might kill herself. She was preoccupied with a worry that she would not be able to get her pension when she reached sixty-five because on a previous hospital admission for diabetes she had used her maiden name when she should have used her married name. She feared that she might be put in jail if this were discovered, and despite reassurance she could not stop talking about it. She was admitted after her sister found her on the kitchen floor after a fall that resulted from weakness because she had not been eating. Physical examination and laboratory tests gave essentially normal results. When interviewed, the patient was agitated, had numerous somatic complaints, and indicated feelings of shame, guilt, and self-disparagement. Her diagnosis was acute depressive reaction. She was referred for electroshock therapy, received twelve treatments, and made a dramatic recovery. She was discharged from the hospital as recovered. (540)

Paranoid disorders. Called paraphrenia in the European literature, paranoid disorders include paranoid states characterized by a well-organized system of paranoid delusions with or without hallucinations and with little or no evidence of intellectual impairment, psychotic paranoid reactions associated with disturbances in intellectual functioning related to chronic brain syndrome, and paranoid symptoms in patients with acute brain syndromes who have underlying paranoid or schizophrenic personality patterns of many years' duration.

Case. Mrs. Palmer, a sixty-four-year-old married woman and a retired saleslady, was brought to the hospital from her home by her two daughters-in-law. They reported that the patient had been "like this" for forty-five years. For several years before admission, she complained frequently of "smelling fumes," of feeling that people were "putting needles into her," that people were trying to break into the house (for this reason, she kept all the doors locked, including the garage door, so that her husband "could not get at the car"). They reported that she had threatened her husband. A son reported that his mother had always been "very emotional, suspicious, and jealous, and a hypochondriac." On admission, the patient was well-oriented and her memory was excellent. She spoke at great length and in great detail, but was guarded and suspicious in her attitude and expressed many of the paranoid ideas reported by her family. Physical examination gave normal findings except for a scar on her left side from an old burn. Her diagnosis was paranoid state superimposed on a paranoid personality of many years' standing. (684)

Other disorders. Miscellaneous disorders without organic brain syndromes, such as personality disorders or situational maladjustments, were classified as "other."

There was not a single case of manic-depressive illness of the manic type, suggesting the rarity of this type of reaction in the elderly mentally ill, although it does occur. Some of the depressed patients evidently had had recurrent depressions even long before the age of sixty, although none had been hospitalized for such an illness prior to age sixty (such patients had been excluded from the sample). Almost three-fourths of the depressed patients had had major physical illnesses requiring hospitalization during the decade preceding the psychiatric illness. At the time of admission, almost one-half had moderate or severe physical disability, although for only four of the thirty-five patients with diagnoses of depression only was physical illness considered to have precipitated the depression.

The symptoms of some of the longstanding schizophrenic patients had been sufficiently well controlled in their younger years that they had not come to the attention of any caretaker who might have had them hospitalized. Some were individuals whose paranoid reaction, usually consisting of fairly well organized delusional systems with little or no evidence of impaired intellectual functioning, began in the involutional period. Some had tended toward increasing isolation and gave evidence of social and personal disorganization, especially certain women who collected increasing amounts of trash, were exaggeratedly penurious, collected animals such as cats or birds in their homes, and showed deterioration in personal habits and appearance. When paranoid manifestations were brief and transient and were considered to be a part of an acute brain syndrome, paranoid disorder was not given as a diagnosis. However, when such symptoms were more persistent and constituted a significant part of the patient's symptomatology, paranoid disorder was noted as a separate diagnosis or as being associated with chronic brain syndrome or affective disorder.

Kay and Roth (1961) have emphasized that "late life schizophrenics" are mostly women and unmarried. Some of them have shown overt paranoid personality patterns all during adult life, but in later life the patterns become more exaggerated and the delusional ideas more evident. The personality remains comparatively well preserved over many years, with little or no evidence of deterioration in intellectual functioning. These investigators consider that there is a strong association between serious physical illness and manic-depressive disorders and between deafness and paranoid reactions. Patients with schizophrenic disorders tend to live as long as the same age group in the normal population.

CHAPTER FOUR

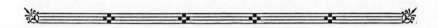

Psychiatric Status

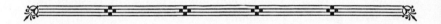

Four indicators of psychiatric status are based on the evaluation and diagnoses made by psychiatrists: the degree of psychiatric impairment at the time of admission; the illness that precipitated admission to the psychiatric screening wards (regardless of accompanying or complicating diagnoses); the differentiation between persons suffering only from organic brain syndromes and those having psychogenic disorders with or without brain syndromes; and the change in degree of impairment during the stay on the screening wards. The fifth indicator of psychiatric status, the number of psychopathological symptoms reported by the patient and/or his collateral informants, and the sixth indicator, orientation to time, place, and person, were gathered by social interviewers when they collected health histories.

PSYCHIATRIC STATUS INDICATORS

Impairment. Most of the elderly patients were rated by reviewing psychiatrists as being severely impaired. The relationship

82

between the assessment of degree of impairment and number of psychopathological symptoms was expected: among the moderately impaired, nearly twice as many patients were reporting only one or no psychopathological symptoms as were reporting six or more (26 per cent, compared with 16 per cent); whereas, among the severely impaired, more than twice as many patients were reporting six or more of these symptoms as were reporting none or only one (34 per cent, compared with 15 per cent). But, as we have pointed out elsewhere (Lowenthal et al., 1967), the relationship is not strong enough to suggest that, even for broad community surveys, the number or type of reported symptoms alone can be used as a basis for classifying a sample according to degree of impairment.

For more than four-fifths of the severely impaired the precipitating condition or primary diagnosis was organic brain syndrome. While most of the moderately impaired patients also had organic brain syndromes, the proportion of psychogenics among them (41 per cent) was considerably greater than among the severely impaired (16 per cent). The dichotomy of any psychogenic disorder versus organic brain syndromes only showed this interrelationship much more dramatically. Thus, 67 per cent of the moderately impaired were classified as having any psychogenic disorder, and 61 per cent of the severely impaired were classified as having organic brain syndrome only. On the test of orientation, the severely impaired were more likely to have been oriented in only one or in no sphere, while the moderately impaired were more likely than not to have been oriented in all three spheres. All subjects who were inaccessible to testing were severely impaired. Finally, no moderately impaired patients deteriorated psychiatrically during their stay on the screening wards. About 80 per cent of both the moderately and severely impaired patients remained the same, and only a handful of the moderately impaired showed more improvement than their severely impaired counterparts. Change on the screening wards was, in general, far more closely related to the type of disorder than to the degree of impairment.

Psychopathological symptoms. A relationship similar to that between the number of psychiatric symptoms and the degree of impairment existed between the scope of reported symptomatology and the admitting diagnosis. Among the 53 per cent whose precipitating condition was acute brain syndrome, the number of reported psychopathological symptoms was quite evenly distributed: just as many had four or more as had less than four. Those for whom the precipitating condition was chronic brain syndrome were more likely to have six or more such symptoms than those suffering from acute brain syndromes (43 per cent, compared with 28 per cent). At the other extreme, those whose precipitating condition was a psychogenic disorder reported somewhat fewer symptoms than those whose precipitating condition was acute brain syndrome (more patients reported four or five symptoms, fewer patients reported six or more). Regardless of the precipitating condition, those patients with any diagnosis of psychogenic disorder had fewer symptoms (only 20 per cent reported six or more) than those with only an organic disorder (39 per cent reported six or more).

The orientation test did not distinguish among the intermediate levels of the symptomatic groups (those reporting two or three; and those reporting four or five), but the level of orientation did show some relationship both to very many and to very few reported psychopathological symptoms: almost three times as many of those reporting none or only one symptom were oriented in all three spheres than were those reporting six or more (43 per cent versus 15 per cent). More than half (56 per cent) of those with six or more symptoms were oriented in only one or none of the three spheres compared to a third (31 per cent) of those with none or only one symptom. Those patients inaccessible to testing were twice as likely to have six or more symptoms than were those with only one or none (34 per cent versus 17 per cent). There was also a relationship between an improvement on the screening wards and the number of reported psychopathological symptoms. More than four times as many of those with one or no such symptoms as those with six or more (30 per cent, compared with 7 per cent) improved on the wards. The proportion of patients whose condition remained unchanged while on the screening wards increased as the number of symptoms increased (from 65 per cent with none or only one symptom to 91 per cent with six or more). A high ranking on the number of symptoms reported did not seem to predict deterioration, but the small number of patients who declined (19) may have obscured a possible relationship.

Precipitating condition. The psychiatric condition that precipitated the patient's admission to the screening wards was moderately assocated with the severity of impairment and with number of reported psychopathological symptoms. This primary diagnosis was also highly correlated with the diagnostic dichotomy of organic brain syndrome only and psychogenic disorder with or without organic impairment. An acute brain syndrome was the major precipitating condition for those in both these groups, but it was more frequent among those only organically impaired (58 per cent) than it was among those with any psychogenic disorder (42 per cent). Among the psychogenically impaired, depression and paranoia, in that order, constituted the next most important precipitating conditions, and among the organically impaired, senile brain syndrome and arteriosclerotic brain syndrome ranked second and third as precipitating conditions. There were marked differences in orientation among the conditions that psychiatrists judged to have precipitated the admission. Patients whose precipitant was either an acute or a chronic brain syndrome were far less oriented than patients whose precipitant was a psychogenic disorder. More than half (53 per cent) of those with chronic brain syndromes were oriented in only one or none of the three spheres of time, place, and person, a quarter were inaccessible to testing, while only a tenth were accessible in all three spheres. Among those with acute brain syndromes, more than twice as many were oriented in only one or none of the spheres than were completely oriented (48 per cent versus 20 per cent). Three-fifths (59 per cent) of persons whose precipitants were psychogenic disorders were completely oriented and only 2 per cent of the psychogenics were inaccessible to testing.

Those whose precipitating condition was acute brain syndrome (53 per cent of the sample) were about three times as likely to change while they were on the screening wards as were those whose precipitating condition was chronic brain syndrome (29 per cent, compared with 11 per cent); even the psychogenics who had no organic brain syndrome did not change as much as those whose precipitating condition was acute brain syndrome. But among those with psychogenic disorders as precipitants, change was more often in the direction of improvement, with a ratio of improvement to deterioration of 22:1, compared with 22:7 among those with acute brain syndrome, and 6:5 among those with chronic brain syndrome as precipitant.

Intellectual functioning. A low level of orientation for this institutionalized sample was closely associated with an admitting diagnosis of chronic brain syndrome, severe psychiatric impairment as indicated by psychiatrists' ratings, and many reported symptoms, while a high level of orientation was associated with an admitting diagnosis of psychogenic disorder, moderate psychiatric impairment, and few psychopathological symptoms. We also noted that there was a correlation between a high level of orientation and improvement during the stay on the ward, but a low level of orientation was not correlated with deterioration (numbers are too small to state this unequivocally). Among those who were considered inaccessible to the orientation test, however, the proportion who deteriorated was more than three times that of those who improved (22 per cent versus 6 per cent). Taking all diagnoses into account and comparing those patients suffering from any psychogenic disorder (with or without brain syndromes) with those patients suffering from brain syndrome only, we found that differences in level of orientation were not as marked as we might have expected. Half (49 per cent) of the psychogenically impaired patients were oriented in all three spheres, while a somewhat greater proportion of the organically impaired patients (58 per cent) were oriented in only one or none of the spheres.

Summary. Another way of reporting the interrelationship among the indicators of psychiatric status is by a measure of association. When the borderline for significant association was set at .16 to .18, most of the indicators were notably interrelated, but the psychogenic/organic diagnostic differentiation attained the best level of association with the other four indicators. The level of orientation was strongly related to the other indicators, especially to that of degree of impairment, to the extent that it was the second best indicator of psychiatric condition. In other words, if, after assigning full and detailed diagnoses, we divided the sample between patients with organic brain syndrome only and those with psychogenic disability with or without an accompanying organic diagnosis, we arrived at a key indicator of psychiatric function and a predictor of short-range prognosis.

Table 9

PSYCHOGENIC/ORGANIC DICHOTOMY BY OTHER
PSYCHIATRIC STATUS INDICATORS

Other Psychiatric Status Indicators	*Psychogenic/Organic Dichotomy*		
	Any Psychogenic	*Organic Only*[a]	*Total*
	%	%	%
Psychiatric impairment			
Moderate	20	7	12
Severe	80	93	88
N	(198)	(266)	(464)

$$\chi^2 = 16.36, \ p < .001, \ v = .19$$

Reported psychopathological symptoms			
None or 1	23	12	16
2 or 3	34	26	30
4 or 5	23	23	23
6 to 12	20	39	31
N	(185)	(278)	(463)

$$\chi^2 = 25.16, \ p < .001, \ v = .23$$

Precipitating condition			
Chronic brain syndrome/ senile brain disease	2	25	16
Chronic brain syndrome/ cerebral arteriosclerosis	2	13	8
Chronic brain syndrome/ alcoholism	5	1	2
Chronic brain syndrome/ other	1	3	2
Acute brain syndrome	42	58	51
Depression	25	--	11
Paranoia	11	--	5
Alcoholic	6	--	2
Character disorder	6	--	3
N	(212)	(293)	(505)

$$\chi^2 = 191.52, \ p < .001, \ v = .62$$

Orientation			
In all 3 spheres	49	7	25
In 2 spheres	21	15	17

Table 9 (Continued)

In 1 or no sphere	25	58	44
Inaccessible	5	20	14
N	(200)	(268)	(468)

$$\chi^2 = 128.91, \; p < .001, \; v = .52$$

Psychiatric change on ward

Improved	32	7	17
Unchanged	64	88	78
Deteriorated	4	5	5
N	(198)	(266)	(464)

$$\chi^2 = 51.44, \; p < .001, \; v = .33$$

[a] Excludes "pure" acute brain syndrome.

PSYCHIATRIC STATUS AND OTHER DOMAINS

Physical condition. Patients with any diagnosis of psychogenic disorder were about twice as likely to be only mildly impaired physically as those with a diagnosis of organic brain syndrome only (24 per cent, compared with 13 per cent); conversely, they were only half as likely to be severely impaired physically (26 per cent, compared with 51 per cent). Patients with psychogenic disorders were about twice as likely to improve physically during the short stay on the screening wards (22 per cent, compared with 12 per cent)' and somewhat less likely to deteriorate than those with organic disorders. Twice as many patients with psychogenic disorders as those with organic disorders had no physical diagnoses (24 per cent versus 12 per cent), while 28 per cent of the latter but only 11 per cent of the former had three or more diagnoses. The other indicators of physical status (the number of reported hospitalizations and the number of reported physical symptoms) showed nearly equal proportions at each level and no trends were apparent. The relationship between the level of orientation and the measures of physical status was similar to that discussed for the psychogenic/organic dichotomy: namely, those oriented in all three spheres were more likely to have been mildly physically impaired and to have had no physical diagnosis, and those inaccessible to testing were more likely to have been severely physically impaired and to have three or more physical diagnoses. Trends were not apparent be-

Table 10

PSYCHOGENIC/ORGANIC DICHOTOMY BY
PHYSICAL STATUS INDICATORS

	Psychogenic/Organic Dichotomy		
Physical Status Indicators	*Any Psychogenic* %	*Organic Only*[a] %	*Total* %
Reported hospitalizations			
None	16	17	16
1	24	30	27
2	23	24	24
3 to 9	37	29	33
N	(172)	(217)	(389)

$$\chi^2 = 2.84, \text{ NS}, \text{ v} = .09$$

Physical complaints			
None or 1	23	25	24
2 or 3	36	29	32
4 or 5	24	24	24
6 to 12	17	22	20
N	(210)	(283)	(493)

$$\chi^2 = 3.16, \text{ NS}, \text{ v} = .08$$

Assigned physical diagnoses			
None	24	12	17
1	44	34	38
2	21	26	24
3 to 6	11	28	21
N	(212)	(293)	(505)

$$\chi^2 = 30.34, \text{ p} < .001, \text{ v} = .25$$

Change in physical condition			
Improved	22	12	16
Unchanged	73	80	77
Deteriorated	5	8	7
N	(171)	(241)	(412)

$$\chi^2 = 9.54, \text{ p} < .01, \text{ v} = .15$$

Note: For the interrelationship between the psychogenic/organic dichotomy and the degree of physical impairment, see Table 13, Chapter Five.

[a] Excludes "pure" acute brain syndrome.

tween the level of orientation and either the number of reported hospitalizations or the number of reported physical symptoms.

Self-maintenance. The relationship between their psychiatric condition and their ability to look after themselves revealed discrete differences between the two diagnostic groups. On every measure of self-maintenance, physical (dressing, eating, bathing, going to the toilet, and so forth) and social (responsiveness, expressiveness, and so forth), patients with psychogenic disorders were considerably more independent. The one item that showed the least difference between the two groups—bathing one's self—suggests that it is something that many organically disordered patients cannot and psychogenically disordered patients will not do for themselves. As one informant for an elderly recluse put it: "No, she doesn't bathe—and won't!" Certainly, the life styles of the Skid Row alcoholics who abound in the psychogenic group result in the scarcity of the proper facilities as well as of motivation. The majority of the psychogenically disordered patients were functioning above the median on all items of self-maintenance, while a majority of the organically disordered were functioning below it on practically all items. The level of orientation, our second best psychiatric indicator, showed a similar pattern in relation to self-maintenance. In every instance, most of the inaccessible patients needed help or were unable to interact effectively with others; most of those who were oriented in all three spheres ranked above the median on all self-maintenance items. The majority of persons oriented in only one or none of the spheres ranked below the median on twice as many self-maintenance items as they did above.

Psychosocial characteristics. Since the average age of the psychogenically disordered patients was 69.5 years and of the organically disordered 77.5 years and, since there were more men among the former (55 per cent) than among the latter (41 per cent), the psychosocial characteristics that distinguished best between the two diagnostic categories were those that can be seen as consequences of the demographic differences. For instance, the proportion of psychogenically disordered patients who lived alone was somewhat greater—in fact, more than half—and we have already noted this to be the pattern for the younger hospitalized males who frequently had an accompanying diagnosis of alcoholism. Then, too, more of the organically impaired patients were widowed, and more of the psychogenically impaired were separated and divorced. This last finding forms a complex of psychosocial difficulties we found in the histories of many of the psychogenic patients (Lowenthal, 1965). They were likely to have records of sporadic employment, psychiatrically impaired family members or histories of losing a parent (usually through death) while they were children. In the light of these past difficulties, the data on recent widowhood (within the preceding ten years) suggested that such losses, although not necessarily precipitating the illness that resulted in the hospitalization, nevertheless added to the vulnerability of these subjects. This was particularly true of the men. Few other psychosocial characteristics distinguished between the two diagnostic groups, but in both diagnostic groups a decline in socioeconomic status since age fifty appeared to be common and a majority of the organically impaired patients were actively involved with a public agency at the time of their admission.

These selected psychosocial characteristics did not markedly distinguish among subgroups of the sample, but it must be remembered that, by the time of the psychiatric examinations, the screening processes of the community and the general hospital had already selected a fairly homogeneous socioeconomic group consisting predominantly of impoverished or economically marginal older people. Consequently many of the psychosocial differences among them were smaller than those separating them from healthier older people in general. With time, however, as the course of disease overwhelmed the patients or was arrested or diminished, some of the characteristics again became important. Marital and present socioeconomic status, for example, had substantial bearing on where these patients were one and two years later.

SUMMARY

Six variables were selected as indicators of psychiatric disability for this sample of aged mental patients: one was derived from reports of psychopathological symptoms, four were derived from a psychiatric examination, and one was derived from results of an orientation test. The interrelationship among the six factors was explored to discover the one that was most closely related to the

Table 11

PSYCHOGENIC/ORGANIC DICHOTOMY BY LOW SELF-MAINTENANCE

	Psychogenic/Organic Dichotomy			
	Psychogenic	*Organic*	*Total*	
Low Self-Maintenance Measures[a]	*Per cent*	*Per cent*	*Per cent*	v
Expression (does not relate experiences)	25	59	45	.33
N	(195)	(277)	(472)	
Toilet (needs assistance)	26	56	44	.30
N	(174)	(254)	(428)	
Money management (does not handle money)	49	76	65	.28
N	(192)	(274)	(466)	
Response (does not respond to questions)	16	41	31	.27
N	(194)	(276)	(470)	
Dressing (dresses for house only)	39	65	54	.26
N	(189)	(267)	(456)	
Quality of social activity (unresponsive to social overtures)	40	67	56	.26
N	(188)	(271)	(459)	

Feeding (needs assistance)	29	49	41	.20
N	(197)	(276)	(473)	
Grooming (partial care of skin, hair, nails)	48	67	59	.19
N	(189)	(264)	(453)	
Safety I (needs hourly safety supervision)	41	60	52	.19
N	(183)	(263)	(446)	
Safety II (needs supervision in same room)	42	60	52	.18
N	(183)	(263)	(446)	
Health (does not care for own health)	42	57	51	.15
N	(196)	(270)	(466)	
Locomotion (cannot manage stairs)	40	55	49	.15
N	(193)	(278)	(471)	
Bathing (does not wash self)	36	48	43	.12
N	(181)	(257)	(438)	

[a] Significance level for the Psychogenic/Organic dichotomy and for each self-maintenance item is $p < .001$, except for Health and Locomotion (each $< .01$), and Bathing ($< .05$).

other five. The dichotomy of any psychogenic or organic brain syndrome only diagnosis proved to have the best degree of association with other indicators. Accordingly, this indicator was used for analysis of the interrelationship of this status with other conditions, status, and circumstances that were called domains: physical condition, self-maintenance, and certain psychosocial characteristics. The level of orientation was also relevant to the baseline psychiatric condition and the short-range outcome. With the variables of the other domains, both the psychiatric status indicators behaved similarly in analysis, which led us to conclude that the type of impairment and the level of orientation may prove useful as convenient screening and predictive tools for the mentally ill of this age group.

When studying short-range changes on the screening wards, we found that those elderly patients who, for psychiatric reasons, were moderately impaired when they were first admitted were no more likely to improve than were the severely impaired; however, only the latter deteriorated; those with acute brain syndromes were the most likely to change, for better or for worse, during their stay on the screening ward, those with chronic brain syndromes were the least likely to change; those with psychogenic disorders were the most likely to improve; those who reported (or had reported for them) few psychopathological symptoms were likely to improve; however, those who reported many symptoms were not likely to deteriorate; similarly, a comparatively high level of orientation status can predict improvement on ward, but a low level of orientation does not necessarily predict deterioration.

CHAPTER FIVE

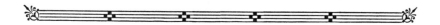

Physical Status

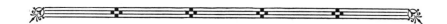

The close relationship between physical condition and mental illness in the elderly has been well documented (Goldfarb, 1961; Dovenmuehle, Newman and Busse, 1960; Gibson, 1961; Kay et al., 1956; Whittier and Korenyi, 1961; Kahn, Goldfarb, Pollack, and Gerber, 1960). Most of our hospital sample patients were seriously in need of physical as well as psychiatric treatment, and a longstanding physical illness was considered by informants to be a condition that, although not sufficient in itself to precipitate hospitalization, was causally associated with the factors that did precipitate hospitalization.

Two of the four measures of physical status that we used are based on information in a health history collected, by social interviewers, from data reported, in most instances, either by the patient or his best informed collateral. The measure comprising the total number of reported hospitalizations is based on the number of surgical and other hospitalizations within the past ten years, but excluded hospitalizations for alcoholic or psychiatric reasons. The measure comprising the total number of reported physical complaints is based on the number of affirmative responses to fifteen questions about physical complaints, asked in terms of past year, and an affirmative response to queries about whether the patient had "ever had a stroke."[1]

The other two measures of physical status are based on individual protocol evaluation by project psychiatrists. In making an evaluation, the psychiatrist consulted the record of physical examination made by the hospital house staff, the patient's hospital chart, and the health history completed by the project's social interviewers. The measure comprising the total number of assigned physical diagnoses is based on the number of diagnoses recorded for each patient and includes both the positive diagnoses and those recorded as "history only" but excludes minor or chronic problems or illnesses such as arthritis, allergies, and hernias.[2] The illnesses occurring most frequently were heart disease and malnutrition, both in 28 per cent of the sample. The incidence of heart disease and of malnutrition are similar to that reported in other studies of aged psychiatric patients (Whittier and Korenyi, 1961, which reported heart disease at 24 per cent; Dovenmuehle, Newman and Busse, 1960, which reported malnutrition at 23 per cent). The degree of physical impairment rating is based on the project psychiatrist's evaluation of functional impairment. The frame of reference is the patient and his disability projected into a hypothetical "standard minimum" environment.[3] A rating of mild impairment implies that it is not

[1] The physical complaints reported for the past year, upon which the physical measure comprising the number of reported complaints is based were: convulsion, fainting, headaches, swelling legs or feet, high blood pressure, stomach problems, bowel condition, skin trouble, "female" trouble, rheumatism/arthritis, falls or injuries, weakness or paralysis in arms or hands, weakness or paralysis in legs or feet, heart or chest pains, kidney or bladder problems, and stroke, the latter not necessarily within the last year.

[2] The physical diagnoses upon which the physical measure comprising the number of assigned physical diagnoses is based were: congestive heart failure, respiratory disease, cerebral vascular accident, malnutrition, diabetes, cirrhosis, cancer, fractures, heart disease, hypertension, peripheral neuritis, moderate or severe hearing impairment, moderate or severe vision impairment, and twenty cases designated as "other," for example, acute barbiturate intoxication.

[3] "Standard minimum environment" is defined as an income ade-

sufficient to interfere with the patient's capacity to maintain himself independently of assistance for daily living. A rating of severe impairment implies total disability. Psychiatrists assigned more weight to certain disorders in the physical system (such as cardiovascular, genito-urinary disorders)' than to impairment in extremities, hearing, and eyesight, and therefore the degree of impairment rating, in its quantitative approach, emphasizes disability.

FOUR INDICATORS OF PHYSICAL STATUS

Hospitalizations. Information on the number of reported hospitalizations in the past ten years was gathered by social interviewers for 76 per cent of the sample. Seventeen per cent had not been in hospital for physical reasons within the preceding ten years. The maximum number of reported hospitalizations was nine. For this analysis, the number of hospitalizations has been grouped into approximate quartiles; none reported, 17 per cent; only one reported, 27 per cent; only two reported, 23 per cent; three to nine reported, 33 per cent. The relationship between the number of reported hospitalizations and the number of reported complaints is significant ($p < .001$) and as expected: persons with many hospitalizations (three or more) were four times as likely to have had many (six or more) complaints (32 per cent) as were persons who had had no hospitalizations (8 per cent). Conversely, fewer complaints (none or one) were reported for persons who had had no hospitalizations (32 per cent) than for persons who had had three or more hospitalizations (6 per cent). There was a tendency for those who had no hospitalizations rather than many to have no

---

quate for basic needs—food, clothing, shelter, essential medical care; no responsibility for care or supervision of another; an urban dwelling unit that made minimal physical demands, such as one that was compact and on one floor, on street level or offered access to street level by elevator, had essential services such as a bath and a telephone, and offered access to essential shopping within easy, level walking distance. Functional disability was determined by an estimate of the amount of supervision required for an individual to live in such an environment. Mild impairment indicates that the subject can live alone but needs limited help during the day with meals, housekeeping, and so forth; moderate impairment indicates that the subject needs to have responsible assistance available most of the time; severe impairment indicates that full-time supervision is required.

physical diagnoses (25 per cent versus 14 per cent). Persons with three or more hospitalizations, however, were no more likely to have three or more diagnoses than were those with none (27 per cent versus 23 per cent). An accumulation of hospitalizations was moderately associated with severe physical impairment. Persons with no hospitalizations were more likely to be rated as mildly impaired physically at the time of admission to the screening wards than were those persons with three or more hospitalizations (28 per cent versus 13 per cent). Those persons with three or more hospitalizations were more likely to be rated as severely impaired (47 per cent versus 34 per cent). The number of hospitalizations during the past ten years, however, had no relationship to change in physical condition while on the screening wards.

Physical complaints. Information about the number of physical complaints was collected by social interviewers for all but 2 per cent of the sample. At least one complaint was mentioned for all but 10 per cent of the patients for whom information was available; the maximum number of complaints mentioned was twelve. The complaints most frequently mentioned were falls or other accidental injuries, weakness of legs or feet, bowel difficulties, rheumatism or arthritis, fainting spells, headaches, and high blood pressure. For this analysis, complaints have been divided into approximate quartiles: none or one complaint, 25 per cent; two or three complaints, 31 per cent; four or five complaints, 24 per cent; and six to twelve complaints, 20 per cent. There is a direct correlation between the number of reported complaints and the number of diagnoses. Four times as many of those patients with six or more complaints were assigned three or more diagnoses as those patients with none or only one complaint (44 per cent versus 11 per cent); the latter were three times as likely to have no diagnoses as those with six or more complaints (27 per cent versus 9 per cent). A similar relationship was found between the number of reported physical complaints and the degree of physical impairment. Persons with few complaints were more likely than those with many to be mildly impaired, while persons with many physical complaints were more likely to be severely impaired. Of the two self-reported health measures, that comprising "many physical complaints in the preceding year" was somewhat more likely to predict severe impairment than was that comprising "many hospitalizations within the past decade," and only the measure comprising the "number of reported physical complaints" was significantly related to both measures based on physicians' evaluation of protocol information. Neither of the measures, however, was related to any change in physical condition while the patients were on the screening wards.

Physical diagnoses. From one to six diagnoses of physical illness were made for 438 of the 534 patients. Eighty-seven patients (17 per cent) received no diagnosis of physical illness, and for nine persons data were not available for assigning a diagnosis. The number of diagnoses was distributed within approximate quartiles: none, 17 per cent; one diagnosis, 37 per cent; two diagnoses, 25 per cent; and three to six diagnoses, 21 per cent.

Just as patients with "few physical complaints" and "few hospitalizations" were mildly physically impaired, and those with "many complaints" and "many hospitalizations" were severely impaired, the patients with many diagnoses were also severely physically impaired. As the number of diagnoses increased, the proportion of persons rated severely impaired increased: 7 per cent with no diagnoses were severely impaired; 31 per cent with one diagnosis, 49 per cent with two diagnoses, and 79 per cent with three or more diagnoses. Sixty-nine per cent of those persons assigned no physical diagnosis were rated mildly impaired, while only one person (one per cent) with three or more diagnoses was so rated. Thus we found an association between the total number of physical diagnoses and two of the other three indicators of physical status. There was also a significant relationship between number of diagnoses and short-term change in physical condition while on the psychiatric screening wards. Persons with none, one, or two diagnoses were much more likely to improve physically than to deteriorate on the wards, while those with three or more diagnoses were as likely to deteriorate as to improve (16 per cent versus 15 per cent). Deterioration on the ward increased with the number of diagnoses: from 2 per cent of those with no diagnosis to 16 per cent of those with three or more.

Physical impairment. On a comprehensive judgment of physical condition at the time of admission to the psychiatric wards, 17 per cent of the hospital sample were rated as mildly physically

impaired, 41 per cent were moderately impaired, and 42 per cent
were severely impaired. These ratings were consistently related to the
other three indicators of physical status. We also found a significant
relationship between the degree of physical impairment and the
change in physical condition while the patients were on the screening wards. None of the persons rated mildly impaired deteriorated
physically while on the screening wards; in fact, all but three of the
persons who did deteriorate were rated severely physically impaired.
There were only slight differences in the proportions of the three
groups that did improve: 10 per cent of the mildly impaired, 19
per cent of the moderately impaired, and 15 per cent of the severely
impaired.

Summary. Of the four measures of the patients' physical
status at time of admission to the psychiatric screening wards, only
the psychiatrist's rating of degree of physical impairment was related
to all other physical measures. Both of the psychiatrist's measures
were more highly associated with each other than they were with
the two measures based on patient or collateral reports, and both
were adequate indicators of the state of general health of the patient
at time of admission to the psychiatric screening wards. The global
degree of physical impairment rating was, however, more closely
associated with short-term change in physical condition than was
number of assigned diagnoses, and we considered it the best indicator of physical condition.

PHYSICAL AND PSYCHIATRIC STATUS

Although in the expected direction, the relationship between
degree of physical impairment and degree of psychiatric impairment
was relatively slight. Physical impairment did, however, have a
marked bearing on the change, particularly any deterioration, in
psychiatric status during the patients' stay on the screening wards.
All but one of the thirty-three persons who deteriorated psychiatrically were rated as severely physically impaired at time of admission.
Conversely, the severely impaired physically were evenly divided
between those who improved and those who deteriorated psychiatrically (11 per cent versus 12 per cent), while among the mildly
or moderately impaired, all but one per cent improved. The degree
of physical impairment measure is not as highly associated with

Table 12

DEGREE OF PHYSICAL IMPAIRMENT BY OTHER PHYSICAL STATUS INDICATORS

Physical Impairment Rating

	Mild %	Moderate %	Severe %	Total N
Reported hospitalizations				
None	28	38	34	(114)
1	23	43	34	(126)
2	10	46	44	(63)
3 to 9	13	40	47	(82)
Total %	20	41	39	(385)

$$\chi^2 = 13.30, \text{ p} < .05, \text{ v} = .13$$

	Mild %	Moderate %	Severe %	Total N
Physical complaints				
None to 1	29	42	29	(100)
2 to 3	19	44	37	(139)
4 to 5	11	43	46	(105)
6 to 12	7	28	65	(74)
Total %	17	41	42	(418)

$$\chi^2 = 32.73, \text{ p} < .001, \text{ v} = .20$$

	Mild %	Moderate %	Severe %	Total N
Assigned physical diagnoses				
None	69	24	7	(67)
1	15	54	31	(162)
2	2	49	49	(105)
3 to 6	1	20	79	(93)
Total %	17	41	42	(427)

$$\chi^2 = 210.66, \text{ p} < .001, \text{ v} = .50$$

Physical Change on Ward

	Improved %	Un-changed %	Dete-riorated %	Total N
Physical impairment				
Mild	10	90	--	(73)
Moderate	19	79	2	(169)
Severe	15	66	19	(176)
Total %	16	75	9	(418)

$$\chi^2 = 45.39, \text{ p} < .001, \text{ v} = .23$$

Table 13

DEGREE OF PHYSICAL IMPAIRMENT BY THE
PSYCHIATRIC STATUS INDICATORS

	Physical Impairment Rating			
	Mild	*Moderate*	*Severe*	*Total*
	%	%	%	%
Psychiatric impairment				
Moderate	22	13	10	13
Severe	78	87	90	87
N	(72)	(174)	(178)	(424)

$$\chi^2 = 7.41, \text{ p} < .05, \text{ v} = .13$$

Psychopathological symptoms				
None or 1	7	19	22	18
2 or 3	35	25	30	29
4 or 5	25	25	21	23
6 to 12	33	31	27	30
N	(69)	(157)	(166)	(392)

$$\chi^2 = 8.52, \text{ NS}, \text{ v} = .10$$

Precipitating condition				
Any chronic brain syndrome	37	33	21	28
Acute brain syndrome only	14	47	72	52
Psychogenic only	49	20	7	20
N	(73)	(175)	(179)	(427)

$$\chi^2 = 90.90, \text{ p} < .001, \text{ v} = .33$$

Organic/Psychogenic dichotomy				
Organic	42	50	74	58
Psychogenic	58	50	26	42
N	(73)	(171)	(168)	(412)

$$\chi^2 = 28.76, \text{ p} < .001, \text{ v} = .26$$

Orientation				
In three spheres	35	34	10	25
In two spheres	19	18	17	18
In one sphere or none	34	38	48	41
Inaccessible	12	10	25	16
N	(68)	(165)	(163)	(396)

$$\chi^2 = 40.13, \text{ p} < .001, \text{ v} = .23$$

Psychiatric change				
Improved	18	21	11	16
Unchanged	82	78	77	78
Deteriorated	--	1	12	6
N	(72)	(174)	(178)	(424)

$$\chi^2 = 33.95, \text{ p} < .001, \text{ v} = .20$$

change in psychiatric status as is the best psychiatric indicator, the dichotomy between psychogenic and organic disorders. However, the relationship between psychiatric diagnosis and psychiatric change while on the ward was accounted for by improvement among the psychogenics, whereas the relationship between degree of physical impairment and psychiatric change was accounted for by deterioration among the severely physically impaired.

Change in physical condition correlated highly with change in psychiatric condition. The majority of those who improved physically improved psychiatrically (58 per cent); none deteriorated. Conversely, the majority of those who deteriorated physically also deteriorated psychiatrically (55 per cent). Correlatons were even stronger the other way around, particularly in regard to deterioration: of those whose psychiatric condition worsened, 78 per cent also deteriorated physically during the stay on the ward. The poorest association was found between the degree of physical impairment and the number of psychopathological symptoms: persons most ill physically had fewer psychopathological symptoms than had the comparatively healthy (22 per cent had one or no psychopathological symptom, compared with 7 per cent of the mildly impaired).

The relationship between the degree of physical impairment and the type of psychiatric disorder is considerably stronger than that between the degree of physical impairment and the degree of psychiatric impairment. Acute brain syndrome must, by definition, be associated with a physiological disturbance (congestive heart failure, malnutrition, alcoholism, and so forth), so it was not surprising to find that more than two-thirds of the severely physically impaired had acute brain syndrome as a precipitating condition. A fifth of the severely physically impaired had a precipitating diagnosis of chronic brain syndrome, and, for half of them, the syndrome was associated with cerebral arteriosclerosis—an expected finding, as a history of stroke is essential to this diagnosis. Almost half of those who were comparatively healthy physically had a psychogenic disorder, mainly depression, as the precipitating condition, and almost one-third had chronic brain syndrome associated with senile brain disease as the precipitating condition. None of the seniles deteriorated physically while on the screening wards (two improved), whereas 15 per cent of those whose primary diagnosis was chronic brain syndrome associated with cerebral arteriosclerosis did so (none improved). As acute brain syndrome is by definition associated with acute physical illness and is potentially reversible if the physiological disturbance responds to treatment, a marked change in the physical health of such patients was expected. Indeed, nearly a third of them did change while on the screening wards: 19 per cent improved; 11 per cent deteriorated, far more than in any other diagnostic group except that with a precipitating condition of alcoholism, where the numbers were too small to permit conclusions (three out of eight improved; none deteriorated).

The mildly and moderately physically impaired were more than three times as likely to have been oriented to time, place, and person as were those who were physically very ill. The severely impaired were somewhat more likely than were the mildly or moderately impaired to have been oriented in none or only one sphere and twice as likely to have been inaccessible to testing. Inaccessible patients tended to deteriorate physically while on the screening ward: 26 per cent deteriorated, 3 per cent improved.

PHYSICAL STATUS AND SELF-MAINTENANCE CAPACITY

In general, all the physical status measures were associated with self-maintenance and the association was as expected, that is, those persons who had favorable ratings on the physical status measures also had favorable ratings on most of the self-maintenance measures, and vice versa. The physical measure most closely associated with self-maintenance was the degree of physical impairment. The majority of the physically impaired were consistently above the median on all items, the moderately impaired on all but two items, the severely impaired on only two of the thirteen items. The degree of physical impairment is significantly related (p < .001) to each of the self-maintenance measures, with severe impairment usually resulting in low self-maintenance. When the measures of self-maintenance were ranked by the measure of association designated as v, locomotion was most highly associated with the degree of impairment, followed by the three primary self-maintenance measures, eating, going to the toilet, and bathing. In general, the relationship between the degree of physical impairment and of self-maintenance was greater than that between the best indicator of psychiatric status (the dichotomy between psychogenic and organic disorders) and self-maintenance. Physical change while on the screening ward was associated with all but two of the self-maintenance items (health supervision and safety supervision in same room) and a greater change occurred in those persons with a low rather than with a high self-maintenance ability. Physical deterioration tended to be correlated with a rank below the median on the self-maintenance items but improvement was not necessarily associated with a high rank, perhaps because there was less opportunity for change.

PHYSICAL STATUS AND PSYCHOSOCIAL FACTORS

The various psychosocial factors were even more weakly associated with physical status than they were with psychiatric condition and the capacity for self-maintenance. Further, the association of psychosocial factors with the strongest indicator of physical impairment (the global ratings) was no greater than with the weaker indicators of physical status (numbers of hospitalizations, of symptoms, and of diagnoses). For example, those persons who were severely physically impaired or who had had three or more hospitalizations during the past ten years were more likely to have been actively involved with a health or welfare agency at the time of admission than were those in better health; persons with many physical diagnoses were likely to have suffered more role loss than those with few diagnoses. Such instances apart, there was little relationship between psychosocial factors and physical condition.

SUMMARY

The physical status measure that was correlated most closely with all the other physical measures was the rating of degree of physical impairment, which was correlated with all the indicators of psychiatric status, except with the number of psychopathological symptoms, and which had a high inverse correlation with all of the self-maintenance measures. Like the other physical indicators, it did not tend to be associated with the various psychosocial measures.

As the best indicator of physical condition at the time of admission, the psychiatrist's rating of degree of impairment may be helpful not only in identifying elderly populations in need of medical assistance, but also in indicating short-term change in the

Table 14

Degree of Physical Impairment by Low Self-Maintenance

| | Physical Impairment Rating | | | | |
Low Self-Maintenance[a]	Mild Per cent	Moderate Per cent	Severe Per cent	Total Per cent	v
Locomotion (cannot manage stairs)	18	41	74	50	.43
N	(71)	(165)	(163)	(399)	
Feeding (needs assistance)	24	29	64	43	.37
N	(70)	(165)	(164)	(399)	
Toilet (needs assistance)	25	31	65	44	.37
N	(65)	(148)	(147)	(360)	
Bathing (does not wash self)	25	33	63	44	.34
N	(65)	(148)	(158)	(371)	
Dressing (dresses for house only)	31	46	72	55	.33
N	(67)	(158)	(163)	(388)	
Grooming (partial care of skin, hair, nails)	37	55	77	61	.31
N	(68)	(155)	(162)	(385)	

Health (does not care for own health)	33	40	68	51	.31
N	(69)	(162)	(165)	(396)	
Expression (does not relate experiences)	33	34	64	46	.30
N	(70)	(166)	(164)	(400)	
Money management (does not handle money)	46	54	80	64	.30
N	(67)	(164)	(164)	(395)	
Social activity (unresponsive to social overtures)	41	33	60	45	.26
N	(69)	(161)	(156)	(386)	
Response (does not respond to questions)	26	21	42	31	.22
N	(70)	(161)	(166)	(397)	
Safety I (needs hourly safety supervision)	21	31	48	36	.22
N	(68)	(155)	(164)	(387)	
Safety II (needs supervision in same room)	37	49	63	53	.20
N	(65)	(154)	(158)	(377)	

[a] Significance level for Degree of Physical Impairment and for each Self-Maintenance item $p < .001$ by chi-square.

patient's physical condition. Neither the number of reported complaints within the past year nor the number of reported hospitalizations within the past ten years related to physical change while on the screening ward. In all but three instances, it was the severely physically impaired who deteriorated physically on the screening wards; of the mildly impaired who changed, all improved. The relationship between the degree of physical impairment and the change in psychiatric condition was accounted for by the fact that the physically most ill deteriorated psychiatrically. Persons with few psychopathological symptoms were likely to improve physically while on the screening wards, but those with many symptoms were not likely to deteriorate. Changes in physical and psychiatric impairment were directly correlated. A rank above the median on the self-maintenance items did not necessarily predict physical improvement, but a rank below the median did tend to predict deterioration.

CHAPTER SIX

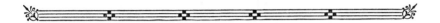

Condition
at Admission
and at Outcome

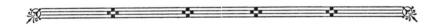

By the first follow-up round of interviewing, more than one-third of the patients in the original sample had died, one-third were in a state hospital, one-quarter were in the community, and 7 per cent were in other facilities, such as nursing homes or the medical wards of general hospitals. Approximately a year later, at the second follow-up, the proportion dead had increased to more than 45 per cent of the sample and the proportion in state hospitals had decreased to 24 per cent. It has been reported frequently in admissions and discharge data that most of the patients who return to the community from state hospitals will have done so within one year after admission. For example, of the first admissions to state hospitals in California who were discharged during the year 1959–60, 88 per cent had been in the hospital for less than a year.[1] For this reason, the first year follow-up location was considered to be the major unit of outcome, and the second year status was used to measure the consistency among the various baseline predictors. Considered as short-range outcomes were the psychiatric change on the ward over a period of only several days and the disposition from the psychiatric screening ward.

AGE AND SEX

Age is closely related to outcome for both the men and the women in the sample. More of the men both improved and declined in psychiatric condition while on the ward, and for both sexes improvement was closely related to age. Thirty-five per cent of the youngest men improved, 18 per cent of the men in their seventies improved, and only 2 per cent of the oldest men improved. The improvement trend for women was similar. Older persons of both sexes were more likely than younger to deteriorate while on the screening wards, but more men than women in each age group deteriorated. Age and disposition from the screening ward are slightly but not significantly related for women. There is very little relation between age and disposition for the men, no doubt largely because the younger alcoholic males were sent from the screening wards to a state hospital. The trend for the women is for fewer to have been released to the community as age increases.

At the first round of follow-up interviewing, we noted a relationship between age and location for both men and women. Forty-four per cent of the youngest men were in the community, 66 per cent of the oldest men had died. Men in the middle age group fell between the youngest and the oldest in the proportions in

[1] Both admissions to state hospitals and the number of people in hospitals have been rapidly decreasing, at least in California, for persons age sixty-five and over. In 1959 (the baseline year of this study), the admission rate for persons sixty-five and over was 236.5 per 100,000 state population; in 1968, the rate had decreased to 89.0. Similarly, in 1959 the rate for the number of persons sixty-five and over in hospitals was 862.6 per 100,000; in 1968, the rate was 221.0 (California Department of Mental Hygiene, 1968).

the community and dead, and were more often found in a state hospital than either of the other two age groups (30 per cent of the seventy to seventy-nine-year-old men were in a state hospital, compared with 24 per cent of the sixty to sixty-nine-year-old men and 17 per cent of the men eighty and older). The relationship between age and location was less apparent for the men by the time of the second round follow-up interview: there was little change among older men, but the proportion dead in the younger age groups increased.

For women, as for men, at the first follow-up interview their age determined whether they were in the community (47 per cent of the younger women) or were dead (42 per cent of the older women). There were no appreciable age differences in the proportions in state hospitals and in other facilities. More women than men at each age level were in a state hospital at the time of the first follow-up interview and fewer were dead. Half as many younger women (13 per cent) as younger men (26 per cent) were dead by the first follow-up interview. As was true for men, the proportion of women deceased within each age group had increased by the time of the second follow-up. Unlike the men, however, this increase was greater for the older age groups (11 per cent, compared with 2 per cent), suggesting, perhaps, that the principle of the "survival of the fittest" holds more true for males than for females.

PSYCHIATRIC CONDITION

Most of the indicators of psychiatric status at the baseline bear a strong relationship to outcome, and, unlike age and sex, they also distinguish among the four categories of disposition.

Psychiatric impairment rating. The global psychiatric impairment rating was less related to outcome than were other psychiatric measures. Indeed, from a strictly statistical point of view, one would not expect a measure with such limited variability (87 per cent were rated severely impaired and 13 per cent were rated moderately impaired) to have very much correlative potential. But, even though the variability of psychiatric impairment is limited, a few more of the patients rated severely impaired than of those rated moderately impaired went to a state hospital from the screening wards, and a few more of the moderately impaired than of the se-

Table 15

OUTCOME MEASURES BY AGE AND SEX

	Men			Women			Total	
	60–69	70–79	80+	60–69	70–79	80+	Men	Women
	%	%	%	%	%	%	%	%
Psychiatric change on ward								
Improved	35	18	2	29	14	2	21	14
Unchanged	59	74	88	70	83	93	71	83
Deteriorated	6	8	10	1	3	5	8	3
N	(83)	(96)	(42)	(69)	(103)	(88)	(221)	(260)
Disposition								
State hospital	68	66	64	71	67	73	67	70
Community	19	16	17	21	16	13	17	17
Other facility	11	13	13	5	16	10	12	11

	2	4	4	1	3	6	5	2
Dead	2	4	4	1	3	6	5	2
N	(281)	(253)	(97)	(109)	(75)	(47)	(109)	(97)
Location at first follow-up								
State hospital	38	26	44	36	34	17	30	24
Community	23	28	6	21	47	6	24	44
Other facility	8	5	8	9	6	11	3	6
Dead	31	41	42	34	13	66	43	26
N	(274)	(245)	(96)	(108)	(70)	(47)	(107)	(91)
Location at second follow-up								
State hospital	29	19	32	28	26	15	22	17
Community	21	26	7	16	47	6	22	40
Other facility	8	6	8	9	6	11	4	7
Dead	42	49	53	47	21	68	52	36
N	(278)	(242)	(97)	(109)	(72)	(47)	(107)	(88)

verely impaired went to the community. By the time of the first
follow-up interview, the degree of initial psychiatric impairment
continued to distinguish between the patients' being in a state hospital or in the community, and proportionately twice as many patients who were rated moderately impaired (12 per cent) were in
other facilities, such as nursing homes, as were patients who were
rated severely impaired (6 per cent). Also, a few more of the severely impaired (36 per cent) than of the moderately impaired (28
per cent) had died. By the time of the second follow-up interview,
the distinction between the moderately and the severely impaired,
in terms of proportions in a state hospital, was negligible, but the
differences in the remaining three location status groups had increased: more of the moderately impaired were either in the community or in other facilities, and more of the severely impaired had
died.

Precipitating condition. Fewer than one-quarter of the patients who had acute brain syndrome or psychogenic diagnosis as a
precipitating condition showed any psychiatric improvement while
on the screening wards; indeed, patients with acute brain syndrome
were more likely to deteriorate. Patients admitted because of chronic
brain syndrome tended to remain in a fairly stable condition while
on the screening wards. Patients with acute brain syndromes were
the least likely to go to a state hospital and the most likely either
to go to another facility or to die. Patients with chronic brain syndromes were the most likely to go to a state hospital, and patients
with psychogenic diagnoses were the most likely to return to the
community. By the time of the first follow-up interview, the relationship between precipitating condition and location status was
much closer and there were shifts in the overall pattern. Compared
with those in the other two diagnostic groups, almost twice as many
patients with chronic brain syndromes were in a state hospital, and
as many patients as in the acute brain syndrome group had died
(43 per cent of the chronic brain syndrome patients and 42 per
cent of the acute brain syndrome patients). There was also a shift
between patients diagnosed as having acute brain syndromes or psychogenic disorders, respectively, in the proportion in other facilities.
By the first follow-up interview, a few more of the psychogenic patients than of the patients with acute brain syndromes were in other

facilities. Only 10 per cent of those patients with any psychogenic disorder had died, while 55 per cent were in the community. By the second follow-up there was little change in this pattern, except that fewer in all diagnostic groups were in a state hospital and more of those with chronic brain syndromes or psychogenic disorders had died.

Multiple diagnoses. More than twice as many patients who received any type of alcoholic diagnosis, regardless of their other diagnoses, improved while on the ward as did patients with only a psychogenic diagnosis, and the latter improved more than did either those with psychogenic and organic diagnoses or those with organic brain syndromes only. Some of the improvement we noticed in the alcoholic group was undoubtedly the result of the clearing of acute brain syndrome associated with alcohol intoxication, and some of the improvement in the psychogenic only group resulted from the clearing of depression after removal from situational stress. There was no marked relationship between multiple diagnoses and disposition except that very few of those diagnosed as having organic brain syndromes only or other chronic brain syndromes (that is, chronic brain syndrome associated with trauma, surgery, and so forth) were released to the community directly from the screening wards.

By the first follow-up interview, the difference in location status among the various diagnostic categories had become marked. Almost half of the patients diagnosed as having organic brain syndromes only had died. Only 11 per cent of them were in the community. This group and those diagnosed as having other types of chronic brain syndrome had the greatest proportion in a state hospital (35 per cent and 53 per cent, respectively). The alcoholics had the next highest proportion in a state hospital (30 per cent), and about one-fourth of the psychogenics only and of those with mixed psychogenic and organic diagnoses were in a state hospital. The psychogenic only patients had the highest proportion in the community (57 per cent) and the lowest proportion dead (7 per cent). There was very little change in the psychogenic group by the time of the second round of follow-up interviewing. The proportion in the community had dropped from 57 per cent to 53 per cent, there was a 2 per cent increase in the proportion in a state hospital and a 2 per cent increase in the proportion who had died. Among the remaining diagnostic categories, the proportions in the community and in other facilities remained about the same, but the proportions in a state hospital dropped from 7 to 11 percentage points, and there was a commensurate increase in the proportion deceased.

Psychogenic diagnosis. The simple dichotomy between any diagnosis of psychogenic illness, regardless of accompanying diagnoses, and a diagnosis of organic brain syndrome only determines location status more sharply than do the other two diagnoses. In fact, this dichotomy was the most powerful predictor of location status of all the measures in the psychiatric domain except for disposition from the psychiatric screening wards. Thirty-two per cent of the patients with psychogenic illness improved while on the ward, whereas 7 per cent of the patients with organic brain syndrome only improved. Proportionately almost twice as many of the psychogenics (23 per cent) as of the organics (11 per cent) returned to the community, and a few more organics were sent to a state hospital. At the time of the first follow-up interview only 10 per cent of the patients with organic brain syndrome only were in the community, compared with 47 per cent of the patients with psychogenic disorders. Proportionately more than twice as many of the former had died, and more than half again as many were in a state hospital. The pattern remained about the same at the second follow-up interview except that the proportion of both the organic brain syndrome only group and the psychogenic group in state hospitals decreased while the proportion that had died, particularly of the organic group, increased.

Psychopathological symptoms. Although the number of psychopathological symptoms was a fair indicator of the short-range outcome, it, and also the psychiatric impairment rating, had the least predictive value at the follow-up rounds. The number of psychopathological symptoms determined those who improved and those who remained the same while on the screening wards; there was very little difference in number of symptoms for those who had deteriorated while on the ward. Of the patients who had one or none of the psychopathological symptoms included in our appraisal, 30 per cent improved, while only 7 per cent of those with six or more symptoms improved.

The proportion of patients sent to a state hospital increased linearly as the number of psychopathological symptoms increased: 53 per cent of those with one or no symptoms, 61 per cent with two or three symptoms, 71 per cent with four or five symptoms, and 84 per cent of those with six or more symptoms went to a state hospital. The proportion of patients who returned to the community was highest for patients with one or no symptoms (22 per cent), but there was no marked decrease with the addition of a few more symptoms (21 per cent of patients with two or three symptoms and 18 per cent of patients with four or five symptoms). However, only 8 per cent of patients with six or more symptoms returned to the community. The highest proportion going to another facility was among patients with the fewest psychopathological symptoms (18 per cent), and the proportional decrease was linear, with 6 per cent of patients with six or more symptoms having gone to another facility. Those patients with the fewest psychopathological symptoms tended to die in greater numbers than patients with more such symptoms (7 per cent of patients with one or no psychiatric symptoms died compared with only 2 per cent among those with six or more symptoms). This is understandable when we remember that those persons with fewest psychopathological symptoms were both more physically impaired and more likely to improve or deteriorate physically on the psychiatric screening ward than were those persons with the most psychopathological symptoms. By the time of the first and second follow-up interviews, the linearity of increase or decrease in proportions of symptoms related to a given location status had all but disappeared, although patients with one or no symptoms were still differentiated from patients with six or more symptoms in being more often in the community and less often in a state hospital. Those patients with the fewest symptoms and those with the most symptoms had a higher death rate than patients with two or three, or four or five symptoms.

Orientation. Orientation was the next most powerful predictor of location status, especially for short-range change, partly because of the association between orientation and psychogenic or organic diagnosis, which was the most powerful predictor of outcome. (The Kent E-G-Y Test, for similar reasons, is also a good predictor of short-range and a powerful predictor of long-range

Table 16

OUTCOME BY BEST INDICATOR IN FOUR DOMAINS

	Domains				
	Psychiatric (Psychogenic/Organic Dichotomy)		Physical (Impairment Severity)		
	Psychogenic	Organic	Mild	Moderate	Severe
	Percentage				
Psychiatric change on ward					
Improved	32	7	18	21	11
Unchanged	64	88	82	78	77
Deteriorated	4	5	-	1	12
N	(198)	(266)	(72)	(174)	(178)
	$\chi^2 = 51.44$, p < .001, v = .33		$\chi^2 = 33.95$, p < .001, v = .20		
Disposition					
Community	23	11	17	22	7
Other institution	9	12	5	4	23

State hospital	66	74	78	74	62
Dead	2	3	-	-	8
N	(212)	(293)	(73)	(175)	(181)

$\chi^2 = 13.52$, p < .01, v = .16 $\chi^2 = 60.52$, p < .001, v = .27

Location at first follow-up

Community	47	10	31	30	15
Other institution	9	5	11	6	7
State hospital	24	39	47	33	26
Dead	20	46	11	31	52
N	(200)	(290)	(72)	(165)	(182)

$\chi^2 = 34.06$, p < .001, v = .46 $\chi^2 = 47.06$, p < .001, v = .24

Location at second follow-up

Community	44	8	29	30	13
Other institution	10	5	10	5	6
State hospital	20	29	40	27	19
Dead	26	58	21	38	62
N	(202)	(293)	(72)	(165)	(182)

$\chi^2 = 33.17$, p < .001, v = .45 $\chi^2 = 45.91$, p < .001, v = .23

Table 16 (Continued)

	Domains				
	Self-Maintenance (Mean, all 13 items)		Psychosocial (Social Living Arrangements)		
	Above Median	Below Median	Alone	With Others	Custodial
	Mean-percentage		Percentage		
Psychiatric change on ward					
Improved	17	15	23	18	4
Unchanged	81	78	72	78	89
Deteriorated	2	7	5	4	7
N	(232)	(203)	(220)	(195)	(71)
	$\bar{\chi}^2 = 6.84$, $p < .05$, $\bar{v} = .12$		$\chi^2 = 13.72$, $p < .01$, $v = .14$		
Disposition					
Community	18	13	20	19	15
Other institution	9	14	13	7	3
State hospital	72	68	64	71	79

(continued)

	(257)	(221)	(238)	(201)	(78)
Dead	1	5	3	3	3

$\bar{\chi}^2 = 9.49$, p < .05, $\bar{v} = .14$ $\chi^2 = 20.55$, p < .01, v = .14

Location at first follow-up

	(242)	(225)	(228)	(199)	(76)
Community	32	17	27	33	4
Other institution	7	7	9	4	9
State hospital	35	31	35	26	38
Dead	26	45	29	37	49

$\bar{\chi}^2 = 23.92$, p < .001, $\bar{v} = .23$ $\chi^2 = 32.00$, p < .001, v = .18

Location at second follow-up

	(243)	(226)	(229)	(200)	(76)
Community	31	15	25	30	3
Other institution	8	7	11	4	5
State hospital	27	22	27	19	30
Dead	34	56	37	47	62

$\bar{\chi}^2 = 26.18$, p < .001, $\bar{v} = .24$ $\chi^2 = 36.53$, p < .001, v = .19

$\bar{\chi}^2$ = mean chi-square of the 13 items (nonadditive).
$\bar{v}$ = mean v score for the 13 items (nonadditive).

outcome.) Thirty-seven per cent of those oriented in all three spheres of time, place, and person improved while on the screening wards, while 9 per cent of those oriented in only one or in no sphere improved. Decline in psychiatric condition, however, was related to whether or not subjects could be tested: 22 per cent of the inaccessible subjects declined compared to 1 to 3 per cent of tested subjects. Orientation also distinguished among the disposition groups: persons oriented in all three spheres were more likely to return to the community, persons oriented in only one or no spheres were somewhat more likely to be sent to a state hospital, persons who could not be tested were likely to be sent to other facilities or to die.

By the time of the first follow-up interview, the proportion of persons who were in the community increased linearly as the level of orientation increased, while the proportion of persons dead increased linearly as the level of orientation decreased. The same pattern prevailed at the second follow-up, with only slight linear decreases in the proportion in the community and somewhat greater linear increases in the proportion dead. Proportionately more persons who were oriented in only one or no spheres were in state hospitals at both follow-up rounds.

PHYSICAL CONDITION

Of the three measures considered in the physical domain, the degree of physical impairment was the best predictor of outcome. While the other two measures, the number of physical diagnoses and the number of physical symptoms, were less related to outcome, their relationship showed much the same pattern as that of the global physical impairment measure.

Physical Impairment. The degree of physical impairment, although not as strong an overall predictor of outcome as psychogenic versus organic diagnosis or as orientation, was more strongly associated with mortality than any measure in the psychiatric, self-maintenance, or psychosocial domains. None of the patients whose physical impairment rating was mild declined psychiatrically while on the ward; 18 per cent improved. Among those patients whose degree of physical impairment was moderate, only 1 per cent declined psychiatrically; 21 per cent improved. Those patients who were severely impaired physically, however, were about as likely to deteriorate psychiatrically (12 per cent) as to improve (11 per cent). There was also very little difference between the mildly and the moderately impaired patients as to disposition from the psychiatric screening wards. None had died, and about the same proportions went to other facilities (5 per cent of the mildly impaired and 4 per cent of the moderately impaired), a few more of the mildly impaired than of the moderately impaired went to a state hospital (78 per cent and 74 per cent, respectively), and a few more of the moderately impaired than of the mildly impaired went back to the community (22 per cent and 17 per cent, respectively). The severely impaired patients had quite different patterns of disposition: 8 per cent died while still on the psychiatric screening wards, 23 per cent went to another facility (in this instance, a medical or surgical hospital for all but three of the forty-two patients), 7 per cent went to the community, and 62 per cent went to a state hospital. By the time of the first round of follow-up interviewing, important differences emerged between the mildly and the moderately physically impaired and the close association between the degree of physical impairment and mortality was even more clear (11 per cent of the mildly impaired, 31 per cent of the moderately impaired, and 52 per cent of the severely impaired had died). Among those who were in a state hospital, the moderately impaired patients occupied a middle position, between the mildly and the severely impaired patients (47 per cent of the mildly impaired, 33 per cent of the moderately impaired, and 26 per cent of the severely impaired were in a state hospital). Among those remaining in the community, there was still no difference between the mildly and the moderately impaired (31 per cent and 30 per cent, respectively), but the proportion was halved (15 per cent) for the severely impaired. Also, at the first follow-up interview, the nature of the other facility had changed from medical to custodial, and more subjects were mildly physically impaired than were severely impaired (11 per cent versus 7 per cent). The relationship, in both strength and kind, that the degree of physical impairment bears to outcome was about the same at the second follow-up interview as it was at the first. The only change was a 6 to 7 per cent decrease in proportions in a state hospital on all levels of physical impairment, and a 7 to 10 per cent increase in proportions deceased on all levels of physical impairment.

Physical symptoms. The short-range outcome, that is the patients' change in psychiatric status while on the screening ward and their disposition, bore little relationship to the number of physical symptoms. Only by the first follow-up interview was there a noticeable though modest association. While the degree of physical impairment was most strongly predictive of death, a paucity of physical symptoms was most closely associated with the likelihood of the patient's being in a state hospital. Forty per cent of patients with no or one symptom were in a state hospital at the time of the first follow-up interview, and only 20 per cent of patients with six or more physical symptoms were there. Thirty-three per cent of the patients with no or one physical symptom and 46 per cent of those with six or more symptoms had died by the first follow-up interview. However, although the relationship between number of physical symptoms and state hospitalization appeared to be linear (that is, patients in the middle range of physical symptoms, two or three, or four or five, fell between those with fewer and those with more physical symptoms in the proportions in state hospitals), this was not the case for patients who had died: the proportion dead among patients with four or five symptoms was lower (29 per cent) than the proportion dead among patients with no or one symptom. We have no definite explanation for the phenomenon, but it suggests that patients suffering from psychiatric or physical impairments must be comparatively healthy to list or complain about the symptoms. It may also be that the patient who complains excessively gets more medical attention than the silent sufferer. The proportions in the community at the first follow-up interview were about 25 per cent in all categories of the numbers of physical symptoms. The pattern at the second round remained essentially the same, and, as was true for degree of physical impairment, there were decreases in the proportions of patients in state hospitals in all symptom groups and concomitant increases in the proportions deceased.

Physical diagnoses. There was very little relationship between the short-range outcome and the number of physical diagnoses. The connection between such diagnoses and any change in psychiatric status was slight and the relationship with disposition from the psychiatric screening wards was modest. Consistent with findings reported by Blau et al. (1962), psychiatric disturbance apparently played a more important role than physical illness in the decision to send a patient from the psychiatric screening wards to a state hospital; at least two-thirds of the patients were so discharged regardless of the number of physical diagnoses recorded. By the first follow-up interview, however, the number of physical diagnoses and the degree of physical impairment predicted death. Nineteen per cent of those patients with no physical diagnosis had died by the first follow-up interview, and the percentages increased linearly, 51 per cent of those persons with three or more diagnoses being deceased. The pattern at the second follow-up interview remained essentially the same. Other than that of death, the best prediction made by the number of physical diagnoses was in the proportions in the community. Thirty-five per cent of the patients with no physical diagnoses were in the community by the first follow-up interview and only 14 per cent of those with three or more diagnoses were. The proportions were almost identical at the second follow-up interview (33 per cent and 13 per cent, respectively).

SELF-MAINTENANCE DOMAIN

All thirteen indicators of self-maintenance tended to be fair predictors of the short-range outcome and to become increasingly important with time. They were, by and large, more closely associated with psychiatric change on ward than were the indicators of physical status, except for degree of physical impairment, and as good or better indicators than were two (impairment severity and precipitating condition) of the five psychiatric indicators. The primary self-maintenance measures predicted disposition from the screening ward better than the physical indicators (again, with the exception of impairment severity) and as well as the indicators of psychiatric status. By the time of the first follow-up, primary self-maintenance measures predicted location status almost as well as did degree of physical impairment, and the secondary self-maintenance measures were even more accurate and proved to be better than, or at least almost as effective as, all the indicators of psychiatric status except that of psychogenic/organic dichotomy. By the

second follow-up they were more effective than all the physical indicators, but still did not come close to the highly effective psycho-
genic/organic dichotomy.

PSYCHOSOCIAL DOMAIN

The psychosocial domain as a whole was much less closely
related to outcome than were the other three domains, though several psychosocial items increased slightly in importance with the
passage of time.

The best indicator of short-term change in the psychosocial
domain (social living arrangements) was not much more powerful
a predictor than the poorest indicator in each of the other domains.
Nor, contrary to our expectations, were any of the measures very
closely associated with disposition from the screening wards. Several
(social living arrangements, complaint-proneness, role status, self-
image) were of some importance as predictors of long-range location status, but none of them was as accurate as the strongest predictors in the other domains. The two psychological factors, complaint-proneness and self-image, emerged, by the time of the second
follow-up, as the most important of the psychosocial items, except
for living arrangements. Patients who were not prone to complain,
or as we interpreted it, were not particularly susceptible to potentially stressful factors were usually back in the community at the
second follow-up. A negative self-image (the information was gathered at the first follow-up interview) was, at the second follow-up,
associated both with death or with being in another facility, primarily medical. Self-image bore no relation to community residence,
but a positive or neutral self-image was strongly associated, at both
follow-up rounds, with being in a state hospital. This suggests that
while the physically ill may suffer from a negative self-image, the
mentally ill do not. We have no way of assessing a possible etiologi-
cal significance to this theory, but perhaps persons with a positive
self-image are prone to mental illness while those with a negative
self-image are more prone to physical illness, or perhaps the mentally ill are not sufficiently aware of themselves to have a negative
self-image.

Whereas living arrangements were not closely associated
with the patients' disposition from the screening wards (those living

alone were somewhat less likely to be sent to state hospitals, those living with others were no more likely to be discharged to the community, those living alone were somewhat more likely to be discharged to another facility) there is a stronger relationship between living arrangements and location one and two years later. Persons who had been living alone or in custodial institutions were more likely to remain in state hospitals (or other facilities) and those who had lived with others had a better chance (better, particularly, than those who had been in custodial institutions) of being in the community. By the time of the first follow-up the proportion of patients who had died increased linearly: 29 per cent of those who lived alone, 37 per cent of those who lived with others, and 49 per cent of those who had been in custodial institutions. There was some increase in this linear relationship at the second follow-up.

SUMMARY

Of the four domains, it was clear that the psychiatric domain, as a whole, had the highest association with outcome. Within this domain, the psychogenic/organic dichotomy was the most closely associated with the patient's change both while on the screening wards and in the long-term, and was only somewhat less associated with disposition than was the degree of physical impairment. Within this domain, orientation was the next best long- and short-range predictor. The self-maintenance domain ranked second to the psychiatric in its association with long-range outcome; the primary self-maintenance measures were more closely associated with short-term change, the secondary self-maintenance measures more closely associated with long-term change. Within the physical domain, the degree of physical impairment rating was somewhat more closely associated with outcome than were the other physical measures. In fact, the degree of physical impairment was more closely associated with disposition from the screening wards than was any other variable in any of the domains. The psychosocial domain as a whole was much less closely associated with outcome than were the other three domains. We found that some of the indicators within the domains predict better than others specific location status at outcome. Patients with a diagnosis of psychogenic disorder, with or without organic brain syndrome, were more likely to have been discharged to the community from both the psychiatric screening wards and from the state hospital; those suffering only from organic brain disease, particularly those with chronic brain syndromes, were more likely to have been discharged from the screening wards to the state hospital. Those with acute brain syndromes were more likely to have been discharged from the screening ward to other institutions or to have died on the ward. By the time of the first follow-up, the organic group was more likely to have died. The best predictor of death, however, both for short-range and long-range outcome, was the degree of physical impairment rating. Age was closely related to outcome for both men and women. The effect of age on location status was strongest for both men and women at the first round of interviewing, when it revealed that the younger patients were in the community and the oldest had died.

If examining physicians are available, the psychogenic/organic dichotomy and the degree of physical impairment obviously have the most prognostic value. But without such evaluations, the self-maintenance measures would make a good second choice. Epstein and Simon (1968) treated the relation between the patients' condition at admission and at outcome with a somewhat different set of measures at outcome.

CHAPTER SEVEN

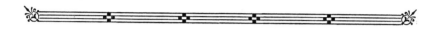

Change in
Patients' Condition

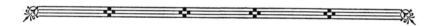

The members of the original baseline sample who were interviewed and reevaluated during the second follow-up comprised the sample studied for changes in the patients' condition. To show the changes that occurred within the widest range of time permitted by our study design, we omitted data from the first follow-up. It will be recalled that during the baseline contact period, staff was located at San Francisco General Hospital. As patients were admitted to the psychiatric wards they were seen by psychiatrists, psychologists, and social interviewers. All patients were interviewed in the same location and in a setting that enhanced the collection of medical data. In addition to interviewing the patients, the social interviewers tried to obtain collateral information from relatives, friends, and any others who might have had additional knowledge of the lives and present circumstances of our subjects. At least one collateral interview was obtained for 486 of the 534 in the original sample, while two collaterals were interviewed for 143 patients, and three were interviewed for twenty. The setting of the collateral interviews varied from a prearranged appointment in a social interviewer's office to an interview on the screening wards or it was frequently a telephone call from the social interviewer to the collateral. Thus, at the baseline interview, there were at least two sources of information about the lives of these patients, and the research schedules often could be completed on the basis of the "best available data," depending on the reliability of the information source in the judgment of the research team. For example, if the patient were in good contact, his own report of self-maintenance activity level was the one recorded, but if the patient were inaccessible, the collateral information was recorded. But by the time of the second follow-up, our subjects were not all in the same place and the research team had moved its offices to the Langley Porter Neuropsychiatric Institute, in another part of San Francisco. Some patients had gone directly from the psychiatric wards to their homes in the community, others were in private hospitals or rest homes, and others were in state hospitals.

Such varying circumstances required changes in the follow-up study design. Because the possibilities for a normal existence are severely curtailed in a state hospital or institutional setting, the social questionnaire developed by the research staff for the initial interview did not seem appropriate for these later interviews. Therefore, two interview schedules were developed. The questionnaire for those in state hospitals or other institutions was limited to the areas of self-maintenance, psychological status, and interviewer ratings. The questionnaire for those in the community covered, in addition, questions about socioeconomic status, social interaction, leisure-time activity, and physical symptoms. There was no attempt to obtain collateral information at the time of the follow-ups because the research staff would be occupied entirely with interviewing patients, who were by this time spread out into rest homes or residences in San Francisco and the Bay Area and in state hospitals in Northern California, so the amount and reliability of information gathered at the second follow-up may be somewhat less than that obtained at baseline, especially for those patients who were in institutions. Patients who were in state hospitals were seen and evaluated by psychiatrists of the research staff, but the psychiatric staff was too small to interview patients who, after two years, were back in the community. Thus, we had medical change data for the patients in state hospitals but not for the rest of the sample.

We measured changes between the baseline and the second follow-up (a period of about two years), by dividing the patients into four groups according to their location at the time of the second follow-up interview. The first location group contained fifty-two patients who were discharged to the community from state hospitals. The second and most varied group consisted of those who were in institutions other than state hospitals; of the thirty-five patients in this group, fifteen were in a county nursing home, eleven were in private rest homes, two each were in private hospitals and in Veterans Administration hospitals, and one each in a medical ward of the San Francisco General Hospital, a private nursing home, a convalescent hospital, a Veterans Administration home, and a boarding home. The third group consisted of thirty-seven patients who were discharged from the psychiatric wards and who were interviewed in the community at the second follow-up. The fourth and largest group included the 125 patients in the state hospitals.

Each patient was counted as belonging to the location group in which he was found at the second-year follow-up. For example, if a patient were discharged to the community from the screening wards, went from his home to a nursing home, from the nursing home back to the screening wards, and from there to a state hospital, where he stayed until he was seen at the time of the second follow-up, he was counted as being in a state hospital. The four groups will be referred to as: the state-hospital, the other-facility, the discharged, and the community groups.

TYPICAL PATIENTS

The following brief sketches illustrate typical patients in each of the groups.

State-hospital patient. The Mother Superior of a tiny Episcopalian convent in the city brought Mrs. Gillafroy to the hospital screening wards on the advice of a social worker. Mrs. Gillafroy, who was eighty-six, had for two years been a lay resident at the convent where she received loving care and attention from her friend, the Mother Superior (who was sixty-five), and two other aging nuns. Since a church ruling forbade the maintenance of such a small convent, it was to be disbanded, so a place had to be found for Mrs. Gillafroy. Although the patient was quite senile upon admission, she had presented relatively few problems for her old guardian sisters. The Mother Superior described her as "very confused" and her memory as "completely gone," and she reported that Mrs. Gillafroy had wandered away from the convent three times during the previous year. The interviewing psychiatrist described this subject as "a classical, sweet Little-Old-Lady who has few intellect resources remaining." In response to most of the questions on the social interview schedule, she merely replied sweetly, "I don't know." Her psychiatric diagnosis was chronic brain syndrome associated with senile brain disease, with no associated physical diagnoses. This patient's admission to the psychiatric wards represents the culmination of a history of senile decline dating back sixteen years prior to her arrival at the hospital. "She started to lose her mind" at the age of seventy, and nine years before admission her second son had her placed in a nursing home. When he died in 1956, she was transferred to a municipal home for the aged. During this period, her only physical difficulties arose from numerous fractures she incurred because of frequent falls. She was sent to Napa State Hospital from the screening wards. When interviewed one year later, she was in a wheelchair with a broken hip. Her demeanor was much as it had been the year before—she smiled sweetly at all the questions—but the irrelevance of her responses clearly indicated severe intellectual impairment. When asked the date, she replied: "Rock Island" or when asked what kind of place she was in, she responded: "Davenport, Iowa." The second follow-up, a year later, revealed that Mrs. Gillafroy, still in a wheelchair, had remained on a steady course. She remained sweet and childlike but was totally incapable of sustaining any response beyond a second or two. When, for instance, she was confronted with an arithmetic problem, she would begin counting on her fingers and then, apparently forgetting the question, would stare incredulously at her arm and hand, muttering all the while incoherent statements of amazement. (380)

Other-facility patient. Mrs. Waterman was brought to the general hospital from the municipal nursing home because she had attempted suicide by trying to jump out of a window. Upon investigation, the research psychiatrist who interviewed Mrs. Waterman learned that she had had an attack of "paroxysmal hypertension and congestive heart failure," causing her to become panic-stricken and hallucinatory ("Those nurses are going around killing people!"). With the arrival of daylight and the administering of medication to control her cardiac symptoms, her panic began to subside, but she remained ruminatively preoccupied with "the things they do to people out there [at the nursing home] at night." Mrs. Waterman was returned to the nursing home from the screening ward because the judge, acting on the Mental Illness Petition, believed her suicide attempt "a fake for the effect it would have upon her son-in-law" [interviewer's notes]. At this remove, it is difficult to justify such a statement, but the record presents a picture of numerous physical diagnoses (pulmonary edema, cardiac heart failure, cystitis in the genito-urinary tract, furunculosis of the skin, and extreme deafness) underlying a moderately acute brain syndrome. The "mildly persecutory" quality in her attention also appears to have had some basis in reality: the death of her daughter within the previous year—a daughter who had cared for Mrs. Waterman —had left her in the home of her son-in-law, who had little love or money for her care. Although she had to be placed in the nursing home on professional medical advice, it does seem that circumstances had conspired to create this special set of misfortunes. Mrs. Waterman was seventy-eight when next seen for the first follow-up interview, which took place in a solarium of the municipal nursing home where Mrs. Waterman had remained since her disposition from the screening wards. Her deafness made interviewing very difficult ("each question had to be shouted directly into her ear"), but her answers were always relevant and, once hearing the question, she responded well. She had made no second attempt at suicide, but it was clear that her poor physical health, her immobility, and the enforced isolation of her deafness were contributing to her low morale. She complained of ward life and the unappetizing food

("They call it a home, but where's the home? It's a barracks, that's all." Indeed her ward contained forty or fifty beds), and she continued to feel a rankling anger at her son-in-law ("I begged him not to send me to this place. He had no right to send me here. Why, my daughter wasn't buried two days before he had another woman in the house"). Fortunately, she was no longer plagued by major physical disabilities—for these she was receiving regular treatment—but the barrenness of her living conditions left her little escape from her brooding. By the time of the second follow-up, a year later, Mrs. Waterman appeared much the same. This time she acknowledged that others probably perceived her as "a crank. Nobody likes me here because I'm so outspoken." Once she became almost tearful when recalling her deceased children, but the interviewer noted that although Mrs. Waterman was "very sad" she was not in "a state of utter despair." "She has a good deal of spunk left," the interviewer added. (643)

Patient discharged from state-hospital. Mr. Chalney, a retired longshoreman, was brought to the general hospital by a representative of his labor union, who had been sent to Mr. Chalney's apartment by the welfare director of the union. The representative found him in a wretched condition: "He hadn't shaved for ten or twelve days, and he had a weird look in his eye." A man who had been sharing quarters with Mr. Chalney was in the process of moving out because of his "peculiar behavior." According to this informant, he had not left the premises "for days on end—felt that people would lock him out." Mr. Chalney was convinced that someone had meddled with the gas range in his kitchen, that people were trying to gas him, and that other people were watching him from another building. The union representative took Mr. Chalney to a nearby health-plan hospital, where he was diagnosed as undernourished, but authorities there recommended the general hospital because of his "mental state." Testing and interviewing this seventy-year-old patient was almost impossible on the screening wards because of his "mute, withdrawn, and suspicious" behavior. Accordingly, his admitting diagnosis was schizophrenic reaction, paranoid type. Three days later, however, he was discharged to a state hospital and there was diagnosed as having a chronic brain syndrome, senile paranoid type. At the state hospital, Mr. Chalney received four electroshock treatments, and within three months his symptoms cleared to the point where he showed insight and partial recall of his earlier difficulties. Consequently, he was discharged on his own cognizance and returned to San Francisco. Mr. Chalney then made several changes in his life: he moved from the apartment house that had been so threatening to him before (a careful check of the facts in this case has shown that Mr. Chalney's charges of exploitation and double-dealing on the part of his landlord were not entirely imaginary). Next, he set up for himself a regimen of a proper diet, daily exercise at home and five- or ten-mile walks through the city, reading, and "inventing activities." To a large extent, these activities were solitary, but this pattern was not inconsistent with a lifetime of aloof, autonomous bachelorhood. Still, if attention were paid him, he enjoyed his relationships with people. The accounts for both follow-up interviews reveal a vigorous and highly articulate man, who was now coping satisfactorily with his life. Although his state hospital experience helped his mental and physical problem, his recollections of the experience were not pleasant: "I don't advise nobody to go there. It's good for some people who are helpless and can't do otherwise—I can't be against that. There are always some unfortunate people who need it, but *I* didn't have to be there!" (636)

Patient discharged to the community.   Mrs. Barish arrived at the county hospital with her husband in a state of agitated, hypertensive depression. According to her husband, she had threatened to shoot herself that morning, but in a collateral interview, he revealed that his wife that "always been nervous and high-strung all of her life. She sounds off and doesn't cater to anyone. Last night she took the cord of the TV set and put it around her neck to choke herself and said she wanted to die." In the previous year, Mrs. Barish had had a "nervous breakdown" following the death of an eighteen-month-old grandchild from "an open spine." She blamed this child's deformity on herself, claiming that the syphilis she had contracted in 1930 had tainted the child. She had been severely depressed ever since this death. Examiners and interviewers noted that Mrs. Barish was oriented and showed no impairment of memory. In fact, "although depressed, she was alert and appeared to be of average or above-average intelligence." A diagnosis of involutional psychotic reaction was given, and the only physical diagnosis was of hypertension. It was recommended that she be transferred to a treatment ward of the general hospital, since the "shock of her admission" to a psychiatric ward appeared to have "toned down her more flagrant symptoms," even though she remained severely agitated, depressed, and capable of only "a tenuous grasp of reality." During her seventy-two-day stay in the hospital, Mrs. Barish received twelve electroshock treatments and participated in some group-therapy sessions. Her later recollections of this experience were unfavorable: she objected to the coercive regimentation of ward life and was somewhat embarrassed by the psychiatric label of her hospitalization, but she was able to acknowledge the great improvement in her physical and mental condition since her discharge. "As I started to feel better, I got to like the routine there a bit better," she said. By the time of the second follow-up interview, Mrs. Barish was again funcioning as the mistress of her household, "clumsily" but affectionately cared for by her husband, and without much situational stress—except for what she considered to be an exorbitant bill for her treatment at the hospital: "I get upset every time I think about it. How am I supposed to get better with that to worry about?" Mrs. Barish impressed the interviewer very favorably: "She seemed a warm and affectionate person, but," she added, "I felt sorry for her. She is a woman who is seldom relaxed. She drives herself to perform what she feels is right in her Christian duty. But, when she gets tired and tense, she becomes so very unhappy that she is unable to do all that she wants or to be the kind of person that she wants to be." (583)

VARIETY OF MOVEMENT

The other-facility group showed the greatest variety of movement as well as the greatest number of moves. Seventeen per cent were in medical hospitals at the second follow-up interview and an additional 34 per cent had been in a medical hospital at least once between interviews. Forty-nine per cent of the other-facility group spent some time in state hospitals and 46 per cent had spent some time in the community. Only one of all the patients interviewed at the second follow-up had been in a private psychiatric facility, and he was a member of the other-facility group. The range of number of moves made was from one to five, with 9 per cent making just one move and 9 per cent making five moves. The modal number of moves was two, and 43 per cent of the other-facility cases fell at the mode. The typical pattern for those who made just two moves (fifteen patients) was an initial disposition to either a state hospital (nine patients) or to the community (five patients) and then to a nursing or boarding home, with just one person going first to a medical hospital and then to a nursing home. The pattern was quite different, however, for those who made three or more moves: fifteen of these seventeen patients spent some time in a medical hospital.

The state-hospital group had the second greatest variety of movement but the least number of moves. Only 6 per cent of this group had been in medical hospitals between interviews (medical need cannot be inferred from this figure as the state hospitals also provide medical services), 12 per cent had been in the community, 8 per cent had been in nursing or boarding homes, and 2 per cent had been in a psychiatric treatment ward at the general hospital.[1] The number of moves made by the state-hospital group ranged from one to seven, and the large majority, 74 per cent, made only one move—directly from the screening wards to a state hospital. Of the thirty-five patients in the state-hospital group who made multiple moves, twenty made three moves, and the typical movement pattern for this group was an initial disposition to the state hospital, an intervening stay either in the community or in a nursing or boardng home, and then readmission to a state hospital. Two of the state-hospital group made as many as seven moves. One of these two patients originally was sent to a medical hospital, then to a county nursing home, back to the medical hospital, on to a state hospital, back to the county nursing home, then to the psychiatric screening wards at the general hospital, and back again to a state hospital where he remained until the second follow-up interview. The other patient originally was committed to a state hospital and then went to the community, from the community to the psychiatric screening wards and back to the state hospital; this pattern was repeated a second time. He provides an excellent example of the pa-

---

[1] These proportions are not additive since three subjects in the state-hospital group were included under two of these location status designations.

tient caught in the revolving door of repeated releases and read-
missions to a state hospital.

> *Case.* Born on a farm in Tipperary, Ireland, Mr. O'Sullivan
> emigrated to the United States in his early twenties. He worked
> as a bartender for almost thirty years, thereby establishing a
> pattern of continuous heavy drinking and "binges" whenever
> his security was threatened. Twice married and divorced, he
> had only one child, a daughter, conceived in the first marriage.
> According to this daughter, Mr. O'Sullivan was a charming,
> hard-working, generous man in his prime: "He liked people
> and people liked him, but drinking has always been his prob-
> lem. I've never been close to him, but I pity him." After re-
> tiring from barkeeping ("I got tired of it and quit"), Mr.
> O'Sullivan took work as a night-watchman in a warehouse.
> Here he sustained an injury to his shoulder that incapacitated
> him, forcing him to retreat from the working world. He sub-
> sequently developed a severe depression that he tried to rem-
> edy with greater quantities of brandy, whiskey, and beer. His
> daughter, visiting him one day from a distant city, persuaded
> him to seek medical treatment for his alcoholism and deteri-
> orated physical condition. Accordingly, Mr. O'Sullivan was
> admitted to the psychiatric wards of the general hospital near
> the end of the baseline year. He was diagnosed as having so-
> ciopathic personality disturbance (alcohol addiction) and gen-
> eralized arteriosclerosis. Mr. O'Sullivan himself requested state
> hospitalization. Within a month, he made a "rapid recovery"
> at the state hospital and was discharged. He impressed the
> social worker at the hospital as being a man who was "very
> realistic about his situation." Upon his return to San Fran-
> cisco, he was reemployed at the warehouse and managed to
> stay "on the wagon" until he again injured his shoulder try-
> ing to wheel a barrow that was too heavy for him. Once
> again, he had to retreat to his one-room apartment for the
> entire day. The old pattern of depression and heavy drinking
> reasserted itself. Within three months, he was back on the
> psychiatric screening wards, from where he was again sent to
> the state hospital. Upon this readmission, he appeared "con-
> fused" and was diagnosed as having a chronic brain syndrome
> associated with alcohol addiction. His physical condition also
> had worsened in the meantime—it was noted that he had de-
> veloped a hemiplegia on the right side of his body. Although
> "cooperative and agreeable," he refused to take any interest
> in group-therapy sessions or Alcoholics Anonymous meetings.

Within a month, he was again discharged and, returned to the city, taking work (at the age of seventy-five) in a funeral home as a janitor and handyman. Mr. O'Sullivan managed to stay out of the hospital this time for six months, but one morning the director of the funeral home discovered him sleeping on the front steps of his establishment and fired him. His daughter found him again, several days later, in his room, badly deteriorated physically and mentally. Once more, he was en route to the state hospital via the screening ward of the general hospital. Upon arrival, he recognized his former refuge ("It's the only place I have"), but was otherwise disoriented and severely impaired physically (arteriosclerotic heart disease). Nine months later, again improved and capable of caring for himself, he was given a leave of absence from the state hospital, but in less than a month, worn out with loneliness, unemployment, boredom, and depression, he returned, totally confused, disoriented, and hyperactive. He was no longer cooperative and seemed to care not at all to relate to the nurses or doctors. The research project was notified in the following year of Mr. O'Sullivan's death in a San Francisco hospital. He died a year to the day after his last readmission to the state hospital. (723)

There was very little variety in the movement of the discharged group and the number of moves was also low considering that this group, by definition, had made at least two moves (namely, a state hospital and the community). Eighty-five per cent of the discharged group moved only between state hospitals and the community and, of these, 86 per cent made this move only once. One patient moved back and forth between a state hospital and the community four times and four patients moved back and forth twice. In addition to the state hospital and the community moves that all patients in this group experienced, 10 per cent spent some time in medical hospitals and 6 per cent spent some time in nursing or boarding homes.

The community group had little movement variety as well as few moves. Fifty-nine per cent of this group went to the community and stayed there, 27 per cent went on to a medical hospital either directly or after an initial stay in the community. Three patients went to psychiatric treatment wards at the general hospital and then returned to the community.

CHANGE AFTER TWO YEARS

Psychiatric status. Change in the psychiatric domain was assessed in relation to the mental status rating and change in WAIS scores. The mental status score was an average of the scores obtained in nine areas of mental functioning: consciousness, orientation, attention, perception, memory, affectivity, idea association, thought quality, and personality and behavior. The possible range of scores within any one of these areas of mental functioning is from 1 (no apparent impairment) through 4 (severe impairment). Psychiatrists and psychologists made the ratings for all patients at the time of the baseline interview but, at the time of the second follow-up, psychiatrists saw only those subjects who were still patients and about half of those were in other facilities. For this reason, the mental status score changes of the state-hospital and other-facility groups are those based on ratings made by psychiatrists, while the mental status score changes of the discharged and community groups are those based on ratings made by psychologists. Although the ratings made by the two disciplines may not be strictly comparable (the percentage of exact agreement between psychiatrists and psychologists on a five-point scale of psychological status at the baseline interview was 61 per cent), ratings made across time within the same discipline are meaningful.

There was very little change in mental status for the state-hospital group. The mean mental status score for this group at the baseline interview was 2.93 and the follow-up score of 2.89 yielded a negligible mean difference of 0.04. Although this slight shift for the state-hospital group is an improvement, more of this group declined than improved (45 per cent improved and 51 per cent declined, for a net decline of 6 per cent; the difference between the larger and smaller proportions of change is the net difference). The apparent discrepancy is owing to the few patients who did improve in relation to the relatively greater degree of deterioration of those who declined.[2] The other-facility group showed significant improvement in their mental status rating. Their baseline score of 2.76

[2] Because the baseline mental status score was 2.93 for the state-hospital group and the lowest possible score was 4.00, the maximum range for improvement was almost twice as great as the maximum range for decline.

Table 17

SUMMARY OF CHANGE BETWEEN BASELINE AND THE SECOND FOLLOW-UP

Domain	*Net Improvement*			
	State Hospital	*Other Facility*	*Discharged or Leave of Absence*	*Community*
	Percentage			
Psychiatric				
Mean mental status rating[a]	−6	79	44	24
WAIS VWS (grouped)	12	59[b]	52	35
Weighted digit span (grouped)	6	33[b]	20	4
Physical				
Number of physical symptoms			39	29
Number of physical diagnoses	11	31		
Specific physical diagnoses:				
Congestive heart failure	0	11		
Respiratory infection	−1	−3		
Stroke	−9	0		
Peripheral neuritis	−2	6		
Malnutrition	23	17		
Diabetes	0	3		
Cirrhosis	0	3		
Cancer	1	(no cases)		
Fractures	−1	0		
Self-Maintenance				
Primary self-maintenance	7	9	75	60
Secondary self-maintenance	−26	4	70	50

[a] At both rounds, the state-hospital and other-facility groups were rated by psychiatrists, the discharged and community groups by psychologists.
[b] Based on N of twenty or less.

Table 17 (Continued)

| | Net Improvement | | | |
	State Hospital	Other Facility	Discharged or Leave of Absence	Community
Domain	Percentage			
Psychosocial				
Religious participation	−15	6	26	0
Role status	−57	−52	−3	−4
Confidant	−24	−18	1	−16
Social interaction			51	50
Organizational activity			18	27
Leisure-time activity:				
TV time			12	38
Radio time			−3	0
Movies			' −5	−9
Reading time			29	0
Social living arrangements:				
Alone both rounds			39	51
With others both rounds			45	37
Changed to Alone[e]			4	9
Changed to With Others[e]			12	3

[e] At the second follow-up.

was slightly better than that of the state-hospital group and they improved significantly over the two-year interval, receiving a mean score of 2.07 at the second follow-up ($\overline{M}$ diff $= 0.67$, t $= 3.51$, p $< .01$).[3] Of the fourteen other-facility patients seen by a psychia-

[3] Tests of statistical significance were used primarily to distinguish turnover from real change. Three tests of significance were used, depending upon their appropriateness to the particular data under consideration. The t test of difference between correlated means (McNemar, 1955, p. 108) was used with interval data that had essentially normal difference distributions. The Wilcoxon Signed-Ranks Matched-Pairs Test (Siegel, 1956, p. 75) was used when data were ordinal and when the amount of change varied. The

trist at the second follow-up interview, eleven had improved and only two declined for a net improvement of 79 per cent. Of the two groups rated by psychologists, the discharged group showed significant improvement; the community group also improved but not significantly. The baseline mean mental status score of the discharged group was 2.03, and the mean score for this group at the second follow-up was 1.73 ($\overline{M}$ diff = 0.30, t = 2.61, p < .02). The community group was better off than the discharged group at the baseline interview, with a mean score of 1.83, but the improvement for the community group in the two-year interval to a mean mental status score of 1.68 ($\overline{M}$ diff = 0.15, t = 1.44, p > .10) was half that of the discharged group. The same picture of improvement prevails for the proportions of improvers and decliners. The net improvement of the discharged group was 44 per cent while the net improvement of the community group was only 24 per cent.

Intellectual status. Intellectual change was assessed by means of four subscales of the WAIS: information, comprehension, arithmetic, and digit span. These subscales were given to all four location groups, but only the change for the total score and for the digit span is reported here because the digit span change is a test of immediate recall and the inability to remember recent events has long been attributed to older persons and to the process of aging (Botwinick, 1967). Both the other-facility and the discharged groups tended to improve their scores on the digit-span test over the two-year period: 50 per cent of the other-facility and 45 per cent of the discharged groups had higher scores at the second follow-up. The net improvement was 33 per cent for the other-facility group and 20 per cent for the discharged group. (The numbers in these groups were reduced because about half of the patients could not be tested at one round or the other, and, because the numbers are small, the reported proportions were not significant.) The amount of digit-span change was high for the community group but just about as many (32 per cent) got lower scores as got higher scores (36 per cent). In the state-hospital group, the modal category was no change (44 per cent), but a few more got higher

---

McNemar test of significance of change (McNemar, 1955, p. 228) was used when the data were categorical.

scores than got lower scores, for a net improvement of 6 per cent.
The changes in the total WAIS score were similar to the changes
in digit span, except that the improvement for the other-facility and
discharged groups was greater (respectively, 67 per cent and 57
per cent improvement), but the community group also showed considerable improvement (52 per cent got higher scores at the second-round interview and 17 per cent got lower scores, for a net
improvement of 35 per cent). The modal category for the state-hospital group was no change, but they had a slightly higher net improvement of 12 per cent.

Physical status. The measurement of physical change among
sample members who survived and those who were interviewed
again after a two-year interval suffers from the same problems as
the measurement of psychiatric change. Medical evaluations of sample survivors who were in the community (both the discharged and
community groups) were not made. However, that group of physical symptoms detailed in Chapter Two was obtained for all sample
members at the baseline interview and for those residing in the
community at the time of the second follow-up. For the state-hospital and other-facility groups, physical diagnoses were made by
project psychiatrists at both the baseline and second follow-up interviews. The physical diagnoses of the other-facility and state-hospital
groups are those that occurred most frequently during the baseline
evaluation and those that were deemed to have the greatest potential consequences for our sample. The diagnoses are: congestive
heart failure, respiratory infection, stroke, peripheral neuritis, malnutrition, diabetes, cirrhosis, cancer, and fractures. Poor vision and
poor hearing have been deleted from change analysis because the
assessment of these defects was qualitatively different each time they
were evaluated. When our patient sample was admitted initially to
the screening ward, glasses and hearing aids were either left home
or removed from the patients upon arrival as a safety precaution.
By the time of the second follow-up, these prosthetic devices had
either been returned or obtained from home for those patients who
had them initially, and some patients had obtained such aids in the
interim.[4]

4 Although the other-facility group was more generally plagued with

Few patients in the institutionalized groups were given any of the nine listed diagnoses during the initial evaluation or changed one way or the other. This, no doubt, is because those who died before the second follow-up had a disproportionate share of such physical problems. As can be seen in Table 17, with the exception of cancer and malnutrition, the other-facility group had more physical diagnoses at the baseline evaluation and tended to improve more than did the state-hospital group. Thirteen per cent of the state-hospital group and 14 per cent of the other-facility group had congestive heart failure initially, and there was no net improvement for the state-hospital group, but the other-facility group showed a net improvement of 11 per cent. Malnutrition—the one diagnosis most amenable to treatment—was also the most frequent diagnosis for both hospitalized groups, but every patient who had malnutrition at the baseline interview had recovered by the second follow-up. None of the change in specific diagnoses was statistically significant, but both groups showed net improvement in terms of the number of physical diagnoses. About half of the other-facility group had fewer diagnoses at the second follow-up, while 18 per cent had more (31 per cent net improvement, significant at less than the .05 level of probability—Wilcoxon Matched-Pairs Signed-Ranks Test). In the state-hospital group, 33 per cent had fewer diagnoses at the second follow-up, but 22 per cent had more, so that the net improvement of 11 per cent was not statistically significant.

The physical differences between these two institutionalized groups reflect differing treatment needs. More of the other-facility group spent some time in medical hospitals, and their physical problems were typically internal, whereas the physical problems of the state-hospital group were typically sensory, and sensory problems are more disruptive of self-maintenance activities such as locomotion, bathing, and responsiveness. The only measure of change in physical condition available for the two groups who were in the community at the time of the second follow-up interview was num-

---

physical problems, the state-hospital patients more frequently had hearing and vision problems (30 per cent versus 14 per cent; precisely, $\chi^2 = 3.27$, 1 df, $p < .10$ for vision problems; while 34 per cent of the state-hospital group compared with only 11 per cent in the other-facility group had problems with hearing, precisely, $\chi^2 = 6.92$, 1 df, $p < .01$).

ber of physical symptoms. The fourteen symptoms were: convulsions, fainting, headaches, swelling in legs and/or feet, high blood pressure, stomach condition, bowel condition, skin trouble, female trouble, rheumatism and/or arthritis, stroke, falls and/or injuries, weakness in limbs, and heart condition. This is essentially the same list as that described in Chapter Two with two minor changes: the kidney and/or bladder trouble symptom is not included here because the question was omitted, inadvertently, from the second-round follow-up health schedule; and the baseline questions on weakness or paralysis in hands and arms and on weakness or paralysis in legs and feet were combined as a question "weakness or paralysis in limbs." Both the discharged and the community groups improved, and had fewer of the reported symptoms at the end of the two-year interval. The mean number of symptoms for the discharged group was 2.92 initially and the mean two years later had fallen by exactly one symptom to 1.92 ($\overline{M}$ diff $= 1.00$, $t = 2.51$, $p < .05$). At the baseline, the community group had a mean of 3.06, slightly more than the discharged group at the time, and the community group also improved, on the average, by one symptom: the community mean number of symptoms at the second round was 2.06 ($\overline{M}$ diff $= 1.00$, $t = 2.67$, $p < .02$). Fifty-eight per cent of both the discharged and the community groups decreased in number of reported symptoms; 29 per cent of the community group increased in number of symptoms compared with only 17 per cent of the discharged group. The net improvement amounted to 39 per cent for the discharged group and 29 per cent for the community group.[5]

Self-maintenance. Ten questions about self-maintenance were selected from the baseline scale of nineteen questions for the second follow-up evaluation. The ten questions have been dichotomized and used to develop two indices, of primary and secondary self-maintenance. The division between primary and secondary was based on whether a given self-maintenance activity was crucial to the immediate health and safety of the patient. The measures of

[5] The apparent discrepancy here (more of the community group declined, yet this group showed a higher level of significant improvement) is owing to the lesser degree of decline and the greater degree of improvement in community subjects.

primary self-maintenance are bathing, feeding, going to the toilet, health supervision, and safety level. The dichotomy for the first three of these items was between the need for assistance and the ability to bathe, eat, or go to the toilet without assistance. Health supervision was divided between those who looked after their own health needs to any extent and those who did not. Safety level was divided between those who could take care of themselves indoors and those who could not. Performance at the higher level on a given item received a score of 1 and the total for the five items formed the index score.

The measures of secondary self-maintenance included dressing, grooming, locomotion, money management, and household activity. Dressing was divided between those who needed some assistance and those who did not; grooming between those who took partial and those who took complete care of their skin, hair, and nails; locomotion between those who could not manage stairs and those who could; money management between those who were not capable of handling money at all and those who were; household activity between those who did housework and those who did not. The secondary self-maintenance index was scored in the same manner. Because of the obvious differences between the four groups in their opportunities for self-maintenance, four of the ten questions were not asked of the institutionalized groups. Two questions—on health supervision and safety level—were omitted from the primary index and two—on locomotion and household activity—from the secondary index. Thus, the range of the indices for the community and discharged groups is from 0 through 5, and the range for the institutional and state-hospital groups is from 0 through 3.

On the primary index, the state-hospital group was maintaining itself at a higher level than the other-facility group at the time of the initial interview. The median index score for the state-hospital group was 1.50 and for the other-facility group was 1.17. Both groups improved slightly more than they declined for a net improvement of 7 per cent for the state-hospital group and 9 per cent for the other-facility group. Secondary self-maintenance, however, presents quite a different picture. The other-facility group was maintaining itself at a slightly higher level than the state-hospital group at baseline (the medians were 1.63 and 1.53, respectively).

The other-facility group stayed at about the same level of functioning (a net improvement of 4 per cent), while the state-hospital group showed significant decline (a net decline of 26 per cent, $z = 2.62$, $p < .01$; all tests of significance for self-maintenance are based on the Wilcoxon Matched-Pairs Signed-Ranks Test). The primary self-maintenance level of the discharged group (median $=$ 3.29) was lower than that of the community group (median $=$ 3.79) at the baseline interview, but the net improvement of the discharged group (75 per cent, $z = 4.66$, $p < .001$) was somewhat better than the net improvement of the community group (60 per cent, $z = 2.61$, $p < .01$). The baseline medians of the discharged and community groups were, however, reversed in the secondary self-maintenance index: the discharged group had a median score of 3.38, while the median score for the community group was 3.00. Even though the discharged group was functioning initially at a higher level than the community group, the discharged still improved somewhat more than the community group. The net improvement of the discharged group was 70 per cent ($z = 4.64$, $p < .001$). The net improvement of the community group was 50 per cent ($z = 3.29$, $p < .002$).

Psychosocial change. Neither the other-facility nor the state-hospital group was particularly active in church—at least when they first became members of our sample. At the baseline round of interviewing, 45 per cent of the other-facility group and 61 per cent of the state-hospital group did not go to church at all, and only 12 per cent of the other-facility and 11 per cent of the state-hospital groups went as often as once a week. The other-facility group showed considerable turnover in religious activity, however: 33 per cent increased their participation and 27 per cent decreased their participation, the net change being a negligible increase of 6 per cent. The state-hospital group, even less active than the other-facility group initially, declined further in the two-year interval. Twelve per cent increased and 27 per cent decreased their participation for a net decrease of 15 per cent ($z = 2.14$, $p < .05$; Wilcoxon Test).

Role status is an index of participation in five roles: those of spouse, parent, organization member, employed person, and church-goer. Two of these roles could not be expected to change very much—those of spouse and parent—and few of the original sample were employed at the time of their admission to the screening wards. However, the remaining roles were subject to considerable change, and for the institutionalized groups, this change was usually a decline. Ten per cent of the other-facility group increased their role status, 62 per cent decreased, for a net decline of 52 per cent ($z = 3.70$, $p < .001$). Among the state-hospital patients, the decline was greater. Seven per cent increased and 64 per cent decreased the number of their roles for a net decrease of 57 per cent ($z = 5.86$, $p < .001$). Intimacy was measured by our asking the patients if they had a confidant, someone with whom they shared personal feelings and problems. Both the other-facility and the state-hospital groups reported a loss of confidants. Twenty-seven per cent of the other-facility group lost a confidant, only 9 per cent gained a confidant; and 35 per cent of the state-hospital group lost a confidant, 11 per cent gained one (state-hospital change: $\chi^2 = 4.05$, 1 df, $p < .05$; McNemar test of significance of change). The same measures of social activity were available for the discharged and community groups. In addition, information was available at both rounds of interviewing for the discharged and community groups about their social interaction, organizational activity, leisure-time activities, and social living arrangements.

The community people, like the institutionalized, were not actively attending church at baseline: 52 per cent did not go to church at all and 20 per cent went to church weekly, and there was very little change in religious participation during the two-year interval between rounds. The same proportion (16 per cent) increased as decreased their church attendance. The discharged group, also relatively inactive at the baseline (56 per cent did not attend church at all and 20 per cent went weekly), did show an increase in church attendance between the baseline and second follow-up interviews. Thirty-one per cent increased and 5 per cent decreased for a net increase in church attendance of 26 per cent ($z = 3.01$, $p < .01$). There was considerable turnover in role status for both the discharged and community groups, but the change was pretty well balanced, with about a third of each group both increasing and decreasing their number of roles (the net change in role status for these groups was a decline of 3 and 4 per cent, respectively). The discharged group was the only group that did not show a decline in intimacy and this also was the group with the highest proportion of confidants at the baseline interview (baseline proportions: discharged, 52 per cent; community, 44 per cent; institutional, 37 per cent; and state-hospital, 14 per cent. These differences were significant by chi-square test at the .01 level of probability). The same proportion (18.5 per cent) of the discharged gained as lost a confidant, while 22 per cent of the community subjects lost a confidant and only 4 per cent gained a confidant. Both the discharged and the community group showed major gains in social interaction. The discharged group had a net increase of 51 per cent ($z = 3.54$, $p < .001$) and the community group had a net increase of 50 per cent ($z = 2.40$, $p < .02$). The two groups also reported an increase in organizational activity. The community group showed the greatest net increase (23 per cent, $z = 1.96$, $p < .05$), with only 4 per cent decreasing. The net increase in the discharged group (15 per cent) was not significant; although the proportion who increased was about the same as in the community group (25 per cent), a few more of the discharged group decreased (10 per cent) their organizational activities. The leisure-time activities of both discharged and community subjects showed some interesting changes. More than 90 per cent of both groups did not go to movies at all at the time of the baseline interview, and those few who changed in the two-year interval went less often. More than half of both groups read for less than an hour a day at the time of the baseline interview, and there was considerable turnover in both groups. Among patients discharged to the community about a third increased and a third decreased, for no net change, but among the discharged group almost two and a half times as many increased as decreased, for a net change of 29 per cent ($z = 2.21$, $p < .05$). At the baseline, less time was spent watching television than was spent listening to the radio. Forty-five per cent of the discharged and 42 per cent of the community group spent more than an hour per day listening to the radio, whereas only 36 per cent of the discharged group and 15 per cent of the community group spent an hour or more watching television. However, by the time of the second follow-up interview, 42 per cent of the community people had increased their television viewing substantially, and only 4 per cent decreased for a net gain of 38 per cent ($z = 2.51$, $p < .02$). Forty-five per cent of the discharged group also increased their television viewing, but many (33 per cent) also decreased and the net gain of 12 per cent was not significant. Radio listening showed a balanced change for both groups with a little more than a third of the discharged and a little more than a quarter of the community groups both increasing and decreasing the time spent listening to the radio. There was not very much change for either group in social living arrangements. About half of the discharged group (51 per cent) lived alone initially and the balance changed to a few more (57 per cent) living with others at the second follow-up interview. Fifty-four per cent of the community group were living alone at the baseline, and this proportion increased to 60 per cent by the second follow-up interview.

PATIENTS' CONDITION AT THE SECOND FOLLOW-UP

The state-hospital group was in worse mental condition than the other-facility group with an average mental status rating corresponding to the "moderate impairment" category, while the other-facility group's score corresponded to "mild impairment." The average mental status scores of the two groups in the community were the same, 1.7, a score between "no impairment" and "mild impairment." However, comparisons between the institutionalized and the community groups are complicated by the fact that psychiatrists rated the institutionalized and psychologists, the community groups. Those in state hospitals had a few more physical diagnoses than did those in other facilities (39 per cent and 24 per cent, respectively, had one or more physical diagnoses). The discharged group had slightly fewer physical symptoms than did the community group (50 per cent, compared with 55 per cent of the community group had two or more physical symptoms).

The institutionalized groups were both at about the mid-point of the zero-to-three scale of primary self-maintenance, indicating that they were able to maintain themselves in half of the three areas of feeding, going to the toilet, and bathing. In the area of secondary self-maintenance, which included dressing, grooming, and money management, the state-hospital patients were, on the average, able to maintain themselves on only one item, while the

Table 18

Condition at the Second Follow-up

	State Hospital	Other Facility	Discharged	Community
Mean mental status rating[a]	2.9	2.1	1.7	1.7
Percentage with one or more physical diagnoses	39	24	50	55
Percentage with two or more physical symptoms				
Mean primary self-maintenance	1.53	1.68	4.76	4.60
Mean secondary self-maintenance	1.13	1.54	4.58	4.54
Percentage with one or more roles	29	41	74	80
Percentage attending church monthly or more	18	39	33	40
Percentage viewing TV more than an hour per day			50	35
Percentage reading more than an hour per day			56	41

[a] At both rounds, the state-hospital and other-facility groups were rated by psychiatrists, the discharged and community groups by psychologists.

other-facility group was at about the midpoint of the scale. The primary self-maintenance scale for the discharged and community groups included two additional items: health supervision and safety level. Subjects in the discharged group were maintaining themselves at a slightly higher level than the community group, who averaged 4.60. Two items were added to the secondary self-maintenance scale for the two groups interviewed in the community: locomotion and household activity. Again, the discharged group was slightly higher than the community group, with a score of 4.54. Although the scale ranges were shorter for the institutionalized group and longer for the groups in the community, it was apparent that the latter were maintaining themselves at a higher level than the former. Both community groups were less than half a point short of passing all items in both scales; the institutionalized groups however barely reached the midpoint on both scales.

The role status of institutionalized patients was considerably lower than that of persons in the community. Twenty-nine per cent of the state-hospital group had one role (neither the state-hospital group nor the other-facility group had more than one role), as did 41 per cent of the other-facility group, while 74 per cent of the discharged group and 80 per cent of the community group had one or more roles. The church attendance of the state-hospital group was considerably lower than that of the other three groups. Eighteen per cent of the state-hospital, 39 per cent of the other-facility, 33 per cent of the discharged, and 40 per cent of the community groups attended church once a month or more often. More of the discharged group than of the community group spent more time in two of our measures of leisure-time activity. Fifty per cent of the discharged and 35 per cent of the community groups spent an hour or more a day watching television, and 56 per cent of the discharged and 41 per cent of the community groups spent an hour or more a day reading.

SUMMARY

The most striking impression resulting from the analysis of change was the apparent appropriateness of the location groups into which the sample was divided. Those who were in the state hospital

were in the worst condition mentally and their physical problems
were few in number, except for loss of hearing and vision. Their
mental condition remained about the same and their physical condition improved slightly. Initially, their primary self-maintenance
was low and there was no net change in the two years between interviews. There was a significant decline in the secondary self-maintenance index. In other words, the state-hospital group maintained
its ability to eat, bathe, and go to the toilet at about the same level
as at baseline, but declined in its ability for grooming, dressing, and
money management. These findings are only partially consistent
with those of Trier (1968), who studied the change in one year of
a continuously state-hospitalized sample drawn from the same original sample as this study.[6] Trier found little change in mental condition, and the slight improvement in sociability that he found is
not corroborated by our findings, although this may be largely the
result of a lack of comparable measures. Trier reported an improvement in the quality of social activity and in response, as well as an
improvement in the psychologist's ratings of cooperation and rapport, although interpersonal behavior declined notably. He attributed these improvements to the patients' having "weathered the
crisis" that led to hospitalization and to the increased social stimulus
of living in a state hospital ward. Our own findings of reduced role
status, loss of intimate relationships, and decline in religious participation, together with Trier's finding of a decline in interpersonal
behavior rating, makes the explanation about weathering a crisis
seem the more likely one. Theoretically, response, cooperation, and
rapport are the more elemental aspects of social behavior upon
which the more complex behavior of intimacy, church-going, and
maintenance roles are built, and it is quite possible that there can
be improvement in the basic elements without the opportunity or
inclination for improvement in the more complex behavior. Also,
because his study focused on change over a one-year period and
ours over a two-year period, the change found by Trier may have

[6] Comparisons between a continuously hospitalized group and a
state-hospital group that includes some patients who moved in and out of
the hospital in the two-year interval should be taken with reservations, although one would think that generally the former group would be in worse
condition.

been a temporary improvement, whereas ours may reflect a secular trend.

The other-facility group was in only slightly better condition mentally than the state-hospital group at the baseline interview, but the other-facility group improved during the two-year interval, whereas the state-hospital group did not. The other-facility group had more physical problems and improved slightly more. At the baseline interview, this group was at a lower level of primary self-maintenance and at a slightly higher level of secondary self-maintenance, and whereas the state-hospital group declined in secondary self-maintenance, the other-facility group improved slightly. The incidence of chronic brain syndromes as precipitants to admission to the screening wards was more than twice as high for the state-hospital group as for the other-facility group (40 per cent and 16 per cent, respectively), with a reverse trend for acute brain syndromes (59 per cent of the other-facility group and 45 per cent of the state-hospital group). An acute brain syndrome is a reversible condition that is associated with a severe physiological disturbance. Both the fact that most of the other-facility group had acute brain syndromes and the fact that more than half of this group spent some time in a medical hospital between the baseline and the second follow-up interviews, suggest that the group's chief problems were physical rather than psychiatric. The changes in intellectual functioning are difficult to interpret. There were substantial gains in all groups except the state-hospital group whose net improvement of 12 per cent was moderate. At the very least, these data do not indicate a decline associated with increasing age or with a progressive brain disease for the sample survivors, but the average scores of this sample are well below those of a sample of normal, aged community residents (Crook and Katz, 1962) and, in this sense, intellectual functioning is certainly related to mental illness in the elderly. Trier also reported an improvement in WAIS scores, and argued that the improvement was the result of a practice-effect. We are inclined to support this view, since an elderly sample psychiatrically hospitalized for the first time would have difficulty responding to this kind of testing, and unlike younger people were almost certainly not exposed to intelligence tests at school. Another possible explanation for the improvement is the better testing conditions during the second follow-up. Although Pierce (1963) found no relationship between testing conditions and WAIS results, his test of this relationship was on the basis of follow-up data because no assessment of testing conditions could be made at the initial interview. (In fact, the assessment of testing conditions was included at subsequent rounds of interviewing because of the original experience of project psychologists who tried to administer tests in the noisy, overcrowded, and frequently disruptive conditions of the screening wards at the baseline interview.) Pierce reported that fifty patients were tested under good conditions in the first re-test, nine were tested under fair conditions, and two under poor conditions. However, if the assessment of testing conditions had been made at the baseline interview, the baseline proportions of good, fair, and poor would be just about the reverse of Pierce's proportions. In addition to these explanations for WAIS improvement, we must note also that the discharged and the other-facility groups, the two with the highest incidence of acute brain syndrome at the time of the initial interview, substantially improved their digit-span scores. This improvement in immediate recall lends some support to the interpretation that it resulted partly from a clearing of the confused state some of the patients were in at the initial interview. In short, it is likely that better testing conditions, a reduction in disorientation and confusion, and possibly some practice-effect all accounted for the improvement of our patients in WAIS scores.

There is good evidence that the state hospital experience was beneficial for the discharged group. In gross terms, patients who were sent to a state hospital and who did not show any mental or physical improvement were still there by the time of the second follow-up interview, but patients who did improve were back in the community. Not only did the discharged group improve, but there is some evidence that they were in better condition than the community group at the time of the second follow-up.[7] The patients

---

[7] A study which analyzed the self-image responses of our hospitalized subjects (Clark, 1963) also found that state hospitalization is not necessarily a destructive experience. She concluded: "In recent years, social scientists . . . have given close attention to the effect of institutionalization *per se* upon the concept of self among the inmates. Conclusions from these studies have emphasized the deleterious effects of the confinement, the regimentation, and the ugliness of 'iron house' living upon patients; but, as we

who had been discharged from the state hospital were not quite as socially active as those discharged from the screening wards to the community, but their mental status was the same, they had slightly fewer physical symptoms and were able to maintain themselves at a slightly higher level. Lowenthal and Trier (1967), in a study of the atttitudes of ex-mental patients, found, contrary to their expectations, that almost half of the discharged sample had positive recollections of their state hospital experience and were in better physical condition than the group of patients who were discharged directly from the screening wards to the community.[8]

---

can see, in the case of our aged mental patients, such generalizations do not necessarily hold. Apparently, institutionalization in itself may provide certain social and personal supports for people who cannot escape the facts of their own dependence. The crucial aspect of social interaction for these mentally ill aged is not confinement or freedom but *the presence or absence of others* [her emphasis] to assist, support, and maintain them through their years of increasing dependence" (p. 13).

[8] The Lowenthal and Trier sample was a one-year follow-up study of the same baseline sample used here.

CHAPTER EIGHT

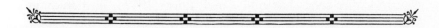

Summary and
Implications

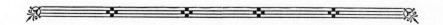

In California the changing policies stimulated by Title XVIII and
Title XIX of the Social Security Amendments of 1965 (Public
Law 89-97) have resulted in a drastic reduction of elderly first
admissions to state hospitals and in the transfer of many elderly
long-term patients to community facilities. As the research of our
colleagues Alvin Goldfarb and Kenneth Jasnau suggests, such alternatives may not be unambiguously better for the patient, or for his
family (Goldfarb, 1962; Jasnau, 1967). What is needed now is a
series of studies of the adjustment of these patients and the course
of their illnesses under a variety of alternative care circumstances,
such as nursing homes, boarding homes, old age homes, and day
care facilities. We believe that such studies will have significance
not only for those suffering from mental illness (in itself often a
fluctuating phenomenon), but for the elderly in general, particu-

larly those in urban centers where increasing ghettolike enclaves heighten fears and anxieties that even under the most serene conditions may accompany the frailties of age. A rhythm of stimulation and tranquility is essential to growth and well-being at all stages of adult life. Older people, sick or well, seem particularly susceptible both to stress and to under-stimulation. An important task for geriatric researchers is to find a way to describe the balance under which those who can no longer independently establish their own rhythms are most likely to thrive, or at worst to survive and then to die with dignity and peace. Our study suggests that in any given year from .5 to 1 per cent of our urban dwellers over sixty will face what initially, at any rate, appears to be a psychiatric crisis, and that most of these will need around-the-clock care or supervision for a few days to several years. They will not only be old and mentally ill but also, most of them, poverty-stricken and physically ill as well.

CONDITION AT ORIGINAL ADMISSION

This group of over five hundred persons confronted with the crisis of psychiatric hospitalization during the first year of the study differed from other San Franciscans over sixty mainly in being economically poorer, living alone, and (even among the youngest males) not having worked for many years. They included proportionately many more women over seventy-five than did the older population in general. Differences were rather minimal in regard to a number of commonly accepted social supports, such as being married, having children in the vicinity, or a religious affiliation. Four-fifths had concerned relatives or friends about them at the time of crisis, and there were no more lifelong isolates or semi-isolates among them than we estimated to exist among elderly San Franciscans in general. Contrary to our hypothesis about age-linked traumas as precipitants, there were relatively few indications of social or psychological stress preceding admission. To be sure, many, in fact a majority, had retired, lost a spouse, or suffered from physical illness or disability, but, for most, these changes had taken place in the distant past, often more than ten years prior to their arrival on the psychiatric screening wards. But they were, on the whole, massively impaired, and many of them had been so for some time.

Psychiatric impairment. In the psychiatrists' judgment, 87 per cent of the patients were severely impaired and in need of twenty-four-hour supervision, and the rest needed considerable care or supervision, though not necessarily around-the-clock. Older subjects were no more likely to be severely impaired than were younger, and men and women tended to be equally impaired, except that women in the middle age range (seventy to seventy-nine) were more ill than either the younger or the older women, and also more ill than men in the same age group. Almost 20 per cent of these patients improved during their screening ward stay (an average of seven days), and only 5 per cent deteriorated. The patients who were relatively younger (under seventy) and especially the men tended to improve while on the screening wards; men also were more likely to deteriorate, and both trends no doubt were partly owing to the greater frequency of acute brain syndromes among men—a condition that is, by definition, temporary and potentially reversible. In fact, the precipitating condition for more than half (53 per cent) of the 525 patients for whom it was possible to assign a diagnosis was acute brain syndrome, the most frequent physical causes of the acute confusional states being malnutrition, congestive heart failure, and alcoholism. The two other principal categories of precipitating condition were chronic brain syndrome (27 per cent) and psychogenic illness (20 per cent), of which depression was the most frequent. Twenty-six patients had attempted suicide just prior to admission, and about half of these had a primary diagnosis of acute brain syndrome, mainly associated with the ingestion of barbiturates.

As a further step in the description of these patients' psychiatric condition, project psychiatrists assigned as many additional diagnoses (up to three) as were relevant. Patients were then grouped into five mutually exclusive diagnostic categories: organic brain syndrome, chronic (arteriosclerotic and/or senile) or acute, but with no accompanying diagnosis of alcoholism or psychogenic disorder (54 per cent); alcoholism, with or without organic brain syndrome (23 per cent); psychogenic disorders, depressive and paranoid, other than alcoholism and without organic brain syndrome (9 per cent); organic brain disorder and psychogenic disorder other than alcoholism (10 per cent); and chronic brain syndrome associated with factors other than senile or arteriosclerotic brain disease (4 per cent).

The psychiatric indicator that correlated best with all other indicators of psychiatric status and with outcome was a division of the diagnostic categories into categories of patients with any psychogenic disorder versus those with organic disorder only, that is, psychogenic disorder with or without accompanying acute or chronic brain syndrome (42 per cent, including alcoholics); and chronic brain syndrome, uncomplicated by psychogenic illness (58 per cent).

Physical impairment. In explaining why the patients were brought to the psychiatric wards, their relatives and other informants mentioned physical health problems in three-fourths of all the cases. The lay appraisals generally were confirmed by project psychiatrists. More than two-fifths of the patients were rated as being severely impaired physically at the time of admission, needing some form of twenty-four-hour care or supervision. Another two-fifths were moderately impaired, that is, had an illness or disability "that definitely limits the patient's capacity to function in some area of everyday living to the degree that he requires some form of assistance or supervision short of twenty-four-hour care." Less than one-fifth were considered mildly impaired. While their physical impairment was not as severe as their mental and emotional impairment, it is obvious that the majority of elderly patients who require emergency psychiatric care in a given year are seriously in need of general medical treatment as well.

More than three-fifths of the patients had been hospitalized for physical reasons during the ten years prior to admission, and one-fourth had had three or more such hospitalizations. This is twice as many as was reported by the community-resident subsample matched with those admitted to the psychiatric screening wards for age, sex, and socioeconomic status. At the time of their admission, about one-fifth were suffering from congestive heart failure, and more than one-fourth showed signs of marked malnutrition (of these, more than a third had a diagnosis of alcoholism). From 8 to 18 per cent had suffered from respiratory disorders, stroke, hearing loss, hypertension, or visual impairment. Lesser health problems or symptoms were numerous: only a tenth had had none at all during the year before hospitalization and almost half had four or more. Physical health problems most frequently reported were, in order of frequency: falls or other accidental injuries, weakness or swelling of legs or feet, bowel difficulties (usually constipation), rheumatism or arthritis, fainting spells, headaches, and high blood pressure. Physical improvement rates during the stay on the screening wards closely resembled those found for psychiatric improvement (those who improved physically were most likely to improve psychiatrically). Predictably, those who improved physically tended to be those who had been admitted for alcoholism, acute brain syndrome, or both, or patients recovering from a suicide attempt with overdoses of drugs. Of all these indicators of physical status, the *degree of impairment* on admission proved to have the highest intercorrelations with other indicators and to be the most strongly associated with the patient's fate one and two years later.

Self-maintenance. In view of their physical and psychiatric condition, the inability of these patients to care for themselves is not remarkable, but it does dramatically illustrate the great stress that their illnesses caused for themselves and others. Lowenthal (1964a), in keeping with the findings of other studies (Blau et al., 1962), emphasized that problems of management and care, rather than reactions to trying or frightening symptoms, played a dominant role in the decisions that took place prior to the patients' admission to the psychiatric wards. Also, the community-resident aged who were psychiatrically impaired differed from hospitalized patients not so much in disturbances of thought, feeling, or behavior, or in the amount or nature of the social supports available to them, as in their capacities for taking care of their own personal needs, being able to dress, select their clothes, take full responsibility for their health, manage money, and, in general, to be self-sustaining (Lowenthal et al., 1967). We suggested that, for elderly people, taking care of one's self may be the functional equivalent of work performance among younger mental patients and ex-mental patients, which is the recovery criterion used by Freeman and Simmons (1963). During the period just prior to admission to the screening wards, half or more of all the patients needed assistance in moving about on more than one level, in grooming or dressing, in handling money, or in looking after their health needs such as special diets, medication, or visits to a physician. Nearly half needed supervision for safety reasons, such as having somebody to make sure stove burners were off or to assist them to cross streets. Two-fifths or more needed help in eating, going to the toilet, and bathing. In measuring their capacity for social interaction we found that, at the time of admission, more than half could not respond to verbal overtures by others, and more than two-fifths could just barely use sentences to make themselves understood. Nearly a third were incapable of any kind of response by word or gesture to simple questions. No single indicator of self-maintenance stands out as being more closely correlated with others, nor is any indicator a markedly better prognosticator than the others. The self-maintenance domain as a whole, however, is very closely related to the patient's subsequent fate. For future screening or research purposes, the number of self-maintenance items could perhaps be reduced, and the results then compared with the key indicators in the psychiatric and physical domains to determine how much and what kind of care the patient needs.

ADMISSION IN RELATION TO OUTCOME

The several domains and indicators clearly differ considerably in the extent to which they are related to the short- and long-range fates of these patients. The type of psychiatric diagnosis, for example, was closely correlated with short-range psychiatric change for better or for worse (while the patient was on the screening wards, an average of seven days), as was the number of reported psychopathological symptoms, whereas the degree of psychiatric impairment at admission was not. There was, however, a strong relationship between the degree of physical impairment and the short-term change in psychiatric condition: those who were seriously ill physically on admission tended to deteriorate psychiatrically, whereas the mildly or moderately impaired physically were more likely to improve psychiatrically. There was a similar pattern for disposition from the screening ward, also a short-range outcome. The type of psychiatric disorder became closely correlated with location one and two years later. The degree of physical impairment at the time of crisis, however, became increasingly significant with time: a severe rating, as might be expected, usually indicated death by the first or second year of follow-up.

The capacity for self-maintenance as measured at the time

of admission to the screening wards is a comparatively good short-term predictor of the patient's fate, and a very good long-term predictor. Nine of the thirteen items used in the self-maintenance scale correlated significantly with changes in psychiatric condition while the patients were on the screening wards, and all thirteen were even more closely correlated with location status at the second follow-up, two years later. Sociocultural factors were negligible predictors of outcome, either long- or short-range. In general, age and sex were more strongly correlated with outcome than were sociocultural characteristics, particularly over the longer time intervals. Age patterns look quite different from the perspective of one or two years. While men at all age levels had a higher mortality rate than women, reflecting trends in the general population, male survivors in the seventy to seventy-nine age group were more likely to be in the community than were women. The women in their seventies appeared to be more vulnerable than younger or older women. By the second follow-up, their mortality rate moved close to that of men the same age, whereas among both the younger and the older women it was considerably lower.

CHANGE IN CONDITION AND OUTCOME

In the discussion of change between the initial assessment and the second follow-up (a period of about two years), the patients were divided into four groups which were based on their location at the time of the second follow-up interview. The groups consisted of fifty-two patients who first went to state hospitals from the screening wards and were then discharged to the community; thirty-five patients who were in institutions other than state hospitals; thirty-seven patients who were discharged from the general hospital psychiatric wards and interviewed in the community at the second follow-up; and 125 patients remaining in the state hospitals. Data for the analysis of change were limited because of variations in coverage between the baseline and the second follow-up (a seemingly unavoidable consequence of personnel changes in research teams). We therefore included all items gathered at both points in time regardless of whether they were included in the other sections of the analysis. We were impressed by the extent to which the analysis of change supported the appropriateness of the second-round location status groups. Those who were sent to and remained in a state hospital were in the worst condition mentally, remaining about the same as at the time of the baseline interview, but there was a slight trend toward physical improvement. Those sent to and remaining in state hospitals also ranked low in primary self-maintenance (activity crucial to the immediate health and safety of the patients) at the baseline, and there was no net change in the two years between the first and last contacts. There was a significant decline in the secondary self-maintenance index, which probably reflects the limited range of opportunities available in state hospitals.

The other-facility group was in only slightly better condition mentally than the state-hospital group at the baseline interview, but improved during the two-year interval, whereas the state-hospital group did not. The other-facility group had more physical problems at the outset and improved slightly more than did those remaining in state hospitals, as they did also in secondary self-maintenance. Patients in this group were far more likely to have been diagnosed as having acute brain syndromes at the time of admission. Since acute brain syndromes have a physical basis, and since more than half of this group spent some time in a general hospital between the baseline and the second follow-up interviews, a picture emerges of a sizeable cohort whose chief problems are more physical than psychiatric. There is evidence that the state hospital experience was beneficial for the discharged group. In gross terms, patients who were sent to state hospitals and who were still in state hospitals did not improve mentally or physically by the time of the second follow-up interview, but patients who were back in the community showed considerable improvement. There is even some evidence that those sent to state hospitals and then discharged were in better condition at the follow-up than the group initially discharged to the community from the screening wards. While not quite as socially active, their mental status was the same as that of the community group, and they had somewhat fewer physical symptoms and were able to maintain themselves at a higher level.

IMPLICATIONS FOR PLANNING AND RESEARCH

Having immersed ourselves in the detailed protocols of these 534 individuals, we have been struck by the overwhelming sense of disintegration that colors these patients' views of themselves, and small wonder, for most of them were indeed very sick, in body, in mind, and no doubt in soul as well. Despair and fear would be the natural reaction to such impairment, at any age. Had they been younger, the influence of the environment in which they found themselves, both before and after admission to the psychiatric screening wards, might well have been less corrosive. The elderly person's conscious or unconscious fear of death, the unknown, is transferred to, or heightens, his fear of another unknown, the institution. This is enhanced by ambivalence toward illness and aging and by the death fears of relatives and friends, and such anxieties in patients and in relatives tend to be stimulated rather than soothed by institutional staffs, who were not only greatly overextended, especially but not exclusively on the screening wards, but also had the problems of their own aging and their own death fears (often triggered by the sight of a helpless older person) despite whatever defenses they might have built up against illness and helplessness. Staff exposure to the aged ill is rarely counterbalanced by personal exposure to elderly persons living under normal circumstances. It is an unfortunate paradox that the rapid urbanization of our society and the increasing geographic segregation or encapsulation of the aged has greatly reduced natural daily contact between young and old, which tempers fear of the unknown with a benign reality, at the very time when nearly all of us can expect to live far beyond sixty. Consequently, the paranoid attitudes, the depression, and the fears of the incapacitated elderly often have some basis in reality (Spence, Feigenbaum, Fitzgerald, and Roth, 1968).

But, what is more important, many on the staffs of our psychiatric institutions, old age, and nursing homes have absorbed, consciously or not, the tacit assumptions of therapeutic nihilism: the person who becomes mentally ill for the first time late in life is suffering from senile (or arteriosclerotic) brain disease, such brain disease is irreversible, therefore this is the end of the road for him. The findings of our research study demonstrate that this assumption is unwarranted. We dealt with the most deprived and the physically most impaired segment of the older urban-resident population, and one that, besides, faced a severely incapacitating psychiatric crisis. To be sure, somewhat more than a third of them died within a year, but they were generally persons who suffered from serious and irreversible physical illness at the time of admission, and were far more likely to be over eighty than under seventy. Yet, after a few days on the screening wards, nearly a sixth of the patients resumed community life; and, of those who were sent to state hospitals, nearly a quarter were able to return to the community within a year. Their physical and psychiatric improvement and their increased capacity to take care of themselves were marked. Even among those who remained in state hospitals, nearly as many improved as deteriorated in several respects.

Impairment, deprivation, and stress. Our hypotheses that age-linked stresses, such as widowhood and retirement, would trigger mental illness and institutionalization were not supported (at least not at the social levels represented by our sample), nor were assumptions connecting a lack of social resources with a greater likelihood of institutionalization. On the contrary, there was some evidence that those discharged from the screening wards to the community had fewer social resources than those sent to state hospitals. This group improved less, on many counts, than that which went to state hospitals and was subsequently discharged. It was the patient's psychiatric and physical condition that most unequivocally influenced his initial fate as a patient, and it was changes in the consequences of those conditions, especially in the capacity for self-care, that were most closely associated with subsequent moves. Despite the overwhelming state of disintegration that these people were in at the time of admission, and despite, for many of them, histories of lifelong deprivation, somewhat more than half survived the period during which we followed them, and well over a third of the survivors were living in the community.

Institutions and alternatives. Many of those who had been in state hospitals and then were discharged seem to have benefited from the experience. Time alone may not have been responsible, but we can only point out that time was not that kind to those who returned to the community directly from the screening wards, and that many patients themselves attributed their improvement to treatment received at the hospital or to other more general social and physical consequences of having been there. That they might have benefited as much or more from different placements is suggested by the follow-up study by Epstein and Simon (1968) of a subsequent cohort of elderly patients who had the advantage of the services of the San Francisco Geriatric Screening Unit team. The fate of the two cohorts of patients suggests that older, like younger, persons may experience periodic crises and, despite their age, their often poor physical condition, and frequently the presence of permanent brain damage, many of the symptoms associated with these crises are reversible or amenable to treatment. The psychiatric improvement that often accompanies comprehensive medical treatment or care strongly indicates the need, long recommended by this research team, for acute psychogeriatric treatment wards, staffed for comprehensive medical care by internists and psychiatrists. The symptoms of neglect found among the marginal group that was discharged from psychiatric screening wards to the community dramatizes with equal forcefulness the need for medical and psychiatric outpatient and supporting community services for the elderly; such services were almost nonexistent at the time of our study and even now are minimal. The remarkable record of the Geriatric Screening Unit team points up two considerations vital for social planning. The first is that mobile teams able and willing to visit prospective patients in their homes can aften alleviate crises before the patient needs to be put in an institution. The second is that nursing home services need to be expanded and, what is even more important, there needs to be a substantial upgrading in the quality and breadth of services offered. One way to accomplish this, apart from establishing and enforcing adequate standards, is with training and education to counteract the outmoded concept of therapeutic nihilism that often characterizes the professional approach to the ill and disturbed aged (Blenkner, 1964). Current mythology to the contrary, not all elderly people who require full-time care in an institution, be it a nursing home, an old age home or a state hospital, are going downhill. For some, the hospitalization in itself becomes a trauma with therapeutic side effects. For others, the shock of transplantation may be a blow from which they do not recover (Blenkner, 1966; Miller and Lieberman, 1965; Lieberman, 1965). For many, this shock could be considerably softened by better communication with the patient and his family about what can be expected and by short-range planning with the patient and his family for specific therapeutic goals, no matter how limited.

There is no doubt that the cumulative stresses of a lifetime have some bearing on psychiatric crises in later life. Although there may be little that the medical and associated professions can do about specific prevention on this score, the concept of the last straw is useful and carries with it implications for treatment. It may be impossible to alter the stressful situations or conditions, but effort can certainly be directed toward reducing strain. This is why an acute treatment unit, whether the presenting symptoms are physical or psychiatric or both, would be especially useful. In such a facility the emphasis would be on getting the individual (and his responsible relatives) over the hump rather than on understanding why he reached the state of crisis. Two considerations, it seems to us, are especially important in this approach: first, an emphasis on relieving physical discomfort (a brief respite of pampering may accomplish miracles) and second, an effort to inform the patient and his family about what realistically to expect. Among older psychiatric patients, the last straw often may be the psychic distress of coping with one more daily round in the face of pain, infirmity, diminished intellectual, affective, and social resources, or sheer frailty. As our companion studies have shown, social amelioratives sometimes may reduce the strains caused by the social losses accompanying aging (loss of income, retirement, or widowhood), but they rarely alleviate the strains of physical illness or incapacity. The chronic disabilities of middle and late life may provide little challenge to the medical profession—the patient is told that these conditions frequently occur in aging persons and he has to "learn to live with it." To the extent that this is the case, the emphasis should be on helping him to live with it, rather than expecting him to bow to fate. In our research and in the work of others, including some dramatic experiments on geriatric wards, it has been demonstrated that almost any kind of support or therapy, whether physical or psychiatric, often will produce astonishing results in functional levels, both physical and psychological. This is not meant to evade the bitter fact that many elderly people who are overcome by a crisis of massive disintegration will die in a year or two, but for the majority of even this most critically afflicted group, short-range therapeutic goals are not only feasible but also can contribute an aura of ritual, dignity, and even purpose to the last phases of life.

Professional roles. It is generally agreed that even a giant computer cannot substitute for the firsthand appraisal of a good clinician. But clinicians are scarce and the elderly population at risk increases and, under such circumstances, next best measures are surely indicated. Our data strongly suggest the feasibility of developing an instrument that can be administered by persons other than physicians to patients and/or their informed collaterals that, with a relatively small margin of false positives or false negatives, could screen out those elderly persons potentially most in need of preventive or therapeutic psychiatric attention. In fact, we developed and pretested such an instrument, which nonprofessionals and professionals can use, before the current analysis was completed (Simon, Berkman, and Epstein, 1968) that appears to be very promising. There seems little question that the prevailing attitude of therapeutic nihilism is partly learned in medical and other professional schools (Spence et al., 1968) and is spread to allied health disciplines and to social planners. Probably only the teaching physician can change this attitude by example and in accordance with known facts. It is to be hoped, too, that in psychiatry and in internal medicine, the teachers will begin to break down their specialist disciplinary barriers when dealing with the elderly, where the interdigitation of psyche and soma becomes dramatically apparent (Lowenthal and Zilli, 1969). The fears and stereotypes of and about the old, whether confounded by illness or not, may be overcome in part by knowledge of the aging process. Thus, medical students, social workers, and nurses, exposed to training in the psychological and sociological aspects of aging, could do much to counteract the prevailing nihilism by coming to understand that the older a person is, the more likely (and with some reason) that accident and illness are occasions for anxiety and panic. But, what is more important, since even chronic illnesses in the very old have their ups and downs, when hospitalization or institutionalization does become necessary neither the patient nor his family should be led to assume that his condition will *necessarily* deteriorate. The idea of temporary short-term treatment, care, and respite, to gather strength to face chronic problems, appears in itself highly therapeutic. The problem of many of the aged is not so much how to face death as how to face life with very real handicaps.

Research. Clearly, before unequivocal recommendations can be made about alternatives to state hospitalization, much more research needs to be done, preferably by assigning such alternatives at random among matched groups of older patients who have psychiatric crises in late life. A screening instrument similar to the one we developed should be administered on a biannual basis over a two-to-five-year period, to check improvement and deterioration under varying circumstances such as state hospitals, nursing homes, old age homes, boarding homes, residence at home assisted by community services, and movement from one to another of these alternatives. Clearly, too, major programs of research should be undertaken on the complex problem of the interrelationship between physical and psychiatric disorder (Lowenthal and Zilli, 1969; Rahe and Holmes, 1966a, 1966b). Such research could perhaps most effectively be carried out within the broader framework of the concept of cumulative stress (Lowenthal et al., 1967). To explore the problem as thoroughly as its importance warrants would require a large community-resident sample, studied at at least two points in time. Such a large scale panel study would also provide an opportunity to explore the marked differences between men and women at successive ages in regard to rates and severity of impairment, and improvement and deterioration over time. Such research should be supplemented by a thorough study of older suicides and attempted suicides, to explore the reasons that the rate for women stays fairly steady at successive ages after midlife, whereas that for men increases sharply with age. Such an analysis not only would help to shed light on age and sex trends, but also should contribute to a better understanding of the complex clinical and social problem of depression in the aged.

Our final recommendation, which could be pursued through a large scale study such as the one just proposed or in smaller studies of all age groups, is for an intensive study of clinical and sub-clinical depression in middle and late life. Our own preliminary findings are that the patterns of association for low morale with, for example, social or physical health, are quite different from the patterns of such association found among those diagnosed as suffering from clinical depression. This suggests that there may be a qualitative rather than a quantitative distinction between the two.

In view of the significant increases in both poor morale and clinical depression with advancing age, a better understanding of their respective etiologies and courses might help to provide a basis for educational and medical preventive programs.

APPENDIX A

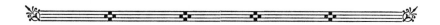

Research Project Committee and Consultants 1958-1959

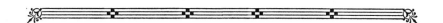

Director, Langley Porter Neuropsychiatric Institute, San Francisco)

ERVING GOFFMAN, Professor of Sociology, University of California, Berkeley (now Professor of Sociology, University of Pennsylvania, Philadelphia)

HAROLD JONES, Late Professor of Psychology, University of California, Berkeley

OSCAR KAPLAN, Professor of Psychology, San Diego State College

MORTON KRAMER, Chief, Biometrics Branch, National Institute of Mental Health (ex officio)

EMMETT B. LITTERAL, M.D., Assistant Superintendent (now Consultant), Agnews State Hospital, Agnews, California

EDWARD S. ROGERS, M.D., School of Public Health, University of California, Berkeley

ELLIS SOX, M.D., Director of Public Health, City and County of San Francisco

NATHAN SLOATE, Chief of Social Service, California Department of Mental Hygiene, Sacramento

RICHARD H. WILLIAMS, PH.D., Chief, Professional Services Branch (now Special Assistant to the Director), National Institute of Mental Health (ex officio)

CONSULTANTS

ROBERT N. BUTLER, M.D., Research Psychiatrist, Study Center, Washington School of Psychiatry, Washington, D.C.

JOHN A. CLAUSEN, Associate Director, Institute of Human Development; and Professor of Sociology, University of California, Berkeley

CHARLES Y. GLOCK, Director, Survey Research Center, and Professor of Sociology, University of California, Berkeley

ALVIN GOLDFARB, M.D., Office of the Consultant on Services for the Aged, New York Department of Mental Hygiene; and Chief, Department of Psychiatry and Neurology, Hospital and Home for Aged and Infirm Hebrews, New York

SAMUEL GREENHOUSE, Chief, Section of Theoretical Statistics and Mathematics, Biometrics Branch, National Institute of Mental Health

WILLIAM E. HENRY, Professor of Psychology, Committee on Human Development, University of Chicago

WAYNE HOLTZMAN, Professor of Psychology (now Dean, College of Education), University of Texas

RICHARD S. LAZARUS, Professor of Psychology, University of California, Berkeley

BENJAMIN Z. LOCKE, Chief, Consultation Section, Biometrics Branch, National Institute of Mental Health

DAVID NASATIR, Instructor of Sociology, University of California, Berkeley

BERNICE L. NEUGARTEN, Professor of Psychology, Committee on Human Development, University of Chicago

TALCOTT PARSONS, Professor of Sociology, Harvard University

HANAN SELVIN, Professor of Sociology, University of California, Berkeley (now Professor of Sociology, University of Rochester)

MARGARET THALER SINGER, Research Psychologist, National Institute of Mental Health

RAMONA TODD, M.D., Senior Physician, Napa State Hospital, Imola, California

PETER TOWNSEND, Professor of Sociology, London School of Economics and Political Science

ROBERT TRYON, PH.D., Late Professor of Psychology, University of California, Berkeley

ANTHONY F. C. WALLACE, Professor of Anthropology, Eastern Pennsylvania Psychiatric Institute

JOSEPH B. WHEELWRIGHT, M.D., Clinical Professor of Psychiatry, University of California, San Francisco

APPENDIX B

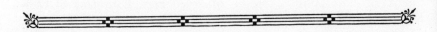

Research Schedules
Used at
Hospital Baseline

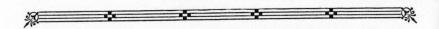

The following schedules were completed for each of the 534 subjects in the Hospital Baseline Sample. N varies for each item within the schedules depending upon whether information was known, refused, and so forth.

Case Summary Sheet. A record sheet filled in by the project secretary. It contains general information on admission and discharge; name, address and telephone number of collaterals; name of interviewers, place and date of interviews.

General Schedule. Some thirteen pages of structured and precoded questions relating to socioeconomic background information, current living conditions including social relationships, work history, and events leading up to hospitalization in the San Francisco General Hospital psychiatric wards. These data were gathered by the social interviewer largely on the basis of "best available information" as elicited from the patient or from collaterals (relatives, friends, and others familiar with the patient and involved in or concerned with admission).

Activity Scale. Consists of fifteen structured categories aimed at the measurement of the subject's level of physical and social self-maintenance at the time it was decided to place him in the San Francisco General Hospital psychiatric ward. Most categories contain items listed in order of decreasing capacity to perform in that category and for each category an entry was made to indicate the length of time that had elapsed since the subject had performed at the highest level. The activity scale ratings were obtained by the social interviewers from the best informed collateral or collaterals.

Health Schedule. A structured instrument used by the social interviewers to record information about a subject's past illnesses and medical care, and some aspects of current physical and psychological health, for example, current state of mind, areas of disturbing behavior. Most data were obtained from "best available information," some, however, were strictly patient-response, collateral-response, or obtained from social interviewer's tests and observations.

Narrative Report of Social Interview. An outline used by the social interviewers in summarizing the steps and reasons leading to admission: description of informant, history of current illness, past medical history, general aspects of the patient's social and economic circumstances and way of life just prior to admission, main events and circumstances of the patient's past life history, his attitudes, values, and future outlook, and the interviewer's observations on the consistency and reliability of the interview materials. This summary was completed for each informant—subject and collateral or collaterals. If information were secured from health and welfare agencies, this was recorded on a separate page for each source.

Medical Data Summary Sheet. The first part of this precoded sheet included demographic data, the official admitting and discharge diagnoses assigned by San Francisco General Hospital staff, disposition, and other medical information gathered by the project secretary from the San Francisco Hospital charts. The second part of the form was used by the project psychiatrist to record his multiple diagnoses, etiology, associated physical diagnoses and other pertinent psychiatric or physical evaluations.

Medical Data Summary Supplement. A precoded form used by the project psychiatrist to record specific physical and neurological findings.

Worksheets Filled in by Examining Psychiatrists. (1) Medical History Summary: a partially structured worksheet used by the psychiatrists to record present illness, systems analysis, past medical history of both patient and family. In addition, the nature, onset, duration, progress, and degree of impairment were recorded. Data were obtained from "best available information," including the health schedule administered by project social interviewers. (2) Mental Status Examination: a worksheet completed by the psychiatrist and based mainly on his observations of the subject's psychological functioning, such as memory and thought quality. Some data were also recorded on specific physical disabilities and general appearance and behavior. (3) Physical Examination Form: a worksheet completed by the psychiatrist. Physical items were indicated as normal or abnormal, and if abnormal, the degree of impairment was noted. Data were derived largely from interns' reports, supplemented by the project psychiatrist's examination when possible. Data from these worksheets were not coded, but were reviewed by psychiatrists when assigned diagnoses and ratings of impairment.

Profile Summary Sheet. A precoded rating form used by the reviewing psychiatrists. Items were rated under the following categories: Activity Level—fifteen items (also recorded by the social interviewer in the Activity Scale) were rated at time of admission on a five-point scale (1, high - 5, low); Psychological Function—items rated on a four-point scale (1, high - 4, low). Two ratings were given for each subject, one at time of admission; one at time of interview; Physical Function—items based on the psychiatrist's various worksheets rated at time of admission on a four-point scale (1, high - 4, low).

Psychological Summary Data Sheet. A sheet upon which the project psychologists entered summary test scores, and ratings of testability and psychological function. They also wrote a brief descriptive paragraph about each subject on this form.

Psychological Rating Data Sheet. On this sheet somewhat more detailed reporting of test results were made (for example, specific WAIS subtest scores, in addition to I.Q.), as well as ratings of psychological functions and impressions of test behavior and attitude.

Ratings of Physical and Psychological Status. A precoded rating sheet used to determine the degree of physical and psychological impairment, each on a five-point scale (0, high - 4, low). Each of the three interviewers—social interviewer, psychologist, psychiatrist—completed this rating immediately after contact with the subject. Use of this form did not begin until halfway through the interviewing year.

Chart Review. A structured form on which Langley Porter residents in psychiatry recorded data abstracted from the San Francsico General Hospital charts, about treatment, laboratory findings, additional physical findings, and nurses' observations. These data provided a basis for rating change in patient's condition during his stay on the screening wards.

FIRST FOLLOW-UP OF HOSPITAL PATIENTS

Schedules were administered approximately one year after baseline. Most of the schedules administered at the first follow-up were identical to or patterned after those used at baseline. Some baseline schedules were combined to form one or part of one first follow-up schedule; others were separated into two parts to fit the interviewing situation of institutionalized and noninstitutionalized. Most of the social interviewers were graduate students in psychology; those who were not were trained to administer psychological tests and therefore acted as both social interviewer and psychologist for this round of follow-up. The number of schedules administered varied because sometimes the interview was not completed (the subject refused to go on, and so on) or the subject died after the social interview but before the psychiatrist's interview, or vice versa.

Case Summary Sheet. This was patterned after the baseline sheet but data recorded here (by the project secretary for each of the 292 subjects remaining in the sample at the first follow-up) pertain to state hospital admission and discharge.

General Schedule. This was patterned after the baseline schedule but some demographic and social items were deleted and others about family and friends were added. Two separate General Schedules were administered: one to subjects who were institutionalized, in a state hospital, nursing home, and so on, at time of interview ($N = 187$); the other to subjects not in an institution at time of interview ($N = 101$). In addition to the items contained in the first schedule, the second contained items on current socioeconomic status, living conditions, and unmet needs.

Activity Scale. Two schedules were administered. The schedule administered to those subjects not institutionalized at the time of interview was identical with the schedule administered at baseline. A different schedule was given to subjects institutionalized at time of interview. It contained the same activity items but was adapted to the institutional situation.

Psychological Summary Sheet. A revised edition included items from both the baseline Psychological Rating Data Sheet and the Psychological Summary Data Sheet. Data were obtained by psychological testing for 277 subjects.

Ratings of Physical and Psychological Status. Identical to baseline form. Rated by social interviewer and psychologists for all subjects seen. (Also rated by the psychiatrists in the Medical Schedule, see below.)

Narrative Report of Social Interview. Although a summary of the interview was again prepared at this round of interviewing, the outline used at baseline was converted to an interviewing schedule and structured questions on plans and expectations, attitudes, values, and self-image were added. Because of the different situations arising from the subject's location at the first follow-up, three different schedules were used: Schedule 1 was used for subjects discharged directly from the San Francisco General Hospital to the community. Schedule 2 was used for subjects discharged or on a leave of absence status from the state hospital. Schedule 3 was used for subjects residing in a state hospital or other institution, for example, nursing home.

Health Schedule. A revised version of the schedule administered at baseline. The data were gathered by the social interviewers or psychologists for ninety subjects who were not in a state hospital at the first follow-up.

Medical Schedule. A new schedule devised at the first follow-up, administered by project psychiatrists to 177 subjects who had entered a state hospital between baseline and the first follow-up (including those who, at time of the interview, had been discharged or were on leave of absence from the state hospital). This schedule contained data modified from the baseline medical forms, all the items from the Health Schedule and new data on reasons for continued hospitalization, state hospital and project psychiatrist's diagnoses, specific physical disabilities, specific geriatric problems, and treatment procedures. In addition, the baseline Medical History Summary worksheet and the Ratings of Physical and Psychological Status were again filled out. Data were obtained from interview and examination of the subject and from the state hospital charts. The psychiatrist also wrote a brief narrative summary of salient points in the schedule, including an overall evaluation of disability and examiner's judgment of the rate and degree of deterioration or improvement and prognosis.

SECOND FOLLOW-UP OF HOSPITAL PATIENTS

Schedules were administered approximately two years after baseline. Interviewers, as at the first follow-up, administered both the social interview and the psychological tests.

Case Summary Sheet. Adapted from the first follow-up sheet and recorded (by the project secretary for each of the 249 subjects remaining in the sample at second follow-up) state hospital admission and discharge information.

Second-Round Schedule for Nonhospitalized Subjects. Administered by the social interviewer or psychologist to ninety-six persons who were not in a state hospital or any other institution at the time of interview. Part of this schedule was adapted from or patterned after the general schedule administered at baseline and the first follow-up. It consisted of short prestructured sections on social and demographic characteristics, psychological and psychopathological symptoms. Baseline health schedule items, psychological tests and a mental status examination were included in the schedule. A prestructured section, patterned after that in the baseline and the first follow-up, was included for psychological ratings and test behavior. A considerable amount of new material was included in the schedule: open-ended questions about stressful conditions and events, pleasant periods, and plans and expectations; precoded Streib and Thompson items, scales 1, 2, and 3 (Thompson, Streib, and Kosa, 1960); a precoded section on drinking patterns and attitudes abstracted from the questionnaire used by the California Drinking Practices Study (Knupfer, 1961); and a precoded section on attitudes that was interspersed with questions from the Srole-Anomie Scale (Srole, 1956). The interviewers also filled out the sheets entitled, *Ratings and Observations of the Subject,* *Ratings of Physical and Psychological Status,* and completed some four pages describing the subject, the circumstances of the interview, and their impressions and interpretations of the interview.

Second-Round Schedule for Hospitalized Subjects. Administered by the social interviewer or psychologist to 151 persons in institutions at the time of interview. This schedule consisted of all material included in the schedule for the nonhospitalized except that no items from the baseline health schedule or the section on drinking were administered. In addition, items from the first follow-up activity scale, adapted to the institutional situation, were included.

Activity Scale. Identical to the activity scale administered at baseline. Data were gathered from ninety-six subjects who were not hospitalized at time of interview.

Narrative Report of Social Interview. Again, a summary of the interview. At this round only one outline was used, patterned after that of the baseline.

Medical Schedule. Patterned after, but more detailed than, the first follow-up medical schedule. The schedule again included all items from the health schedule and the *Ratings of Physical and Psychological Status.* The schedule was administered by the psychiatrist to subjects in state hospitals, those discharged or on leave of absence from state hospitals, and those residing in another institution at time of interview (N = 157).

History of Illness Schedule. Basically a life history summary in structured form for recording, case-by-case, the development of every psychiatric symptom, the time it appeared, environmental changes, psychological changes, social changes, and the dates that these changes occurred throughout the patient's life. This was to show in condensed form the sequence in which illnesses and related conditions occurred. Psychiatric social workers, who were specifically recruited to handle this task, and Langley Porter residents in psychiatry recorded these data from project records, from state hospital charts, and from San Francisco General Hospital charts. As well as providing a convenient form for case reviews by clinicians, these schedules, coded in selected global terms, provided the basis for an analysis of sequences of events or changes in the patients' lives.

APPENDIX C

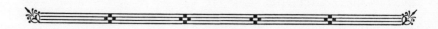

Accessibility Scale

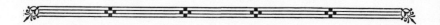

Of the 534 patients who constituted the hospital baseline sample, 502 were seen by a social interviewer. Some of the patients responded quite well to the interview and others were completely unable to respond. The uncommunicative patients we called the Inaccessibles. In the baseline General Schedule (see Appendix B) were fourteen questions that were asked only of the patients and not of the collaterals. The number of patients coded as Inaccessible on any of these fourteen questions ranged from 175 to 228. Not all of the patients were completely inaccessible, however, and in order to describe inaccessibility briefly, the hospital sample was stratified on a scale of accessibility and compared on the variables of age, sex, present socioeconomic status, rank on the Social and the Physical Self-Maintenance Scales, diagnosis, and location one year after the first admission.

The Accessibility Scale is part of a coding document developed by Helen Jambor and Joe Spaeth in August 1960. A Narrative Report was written by the social interviewer for each patient and/or collateral interviewed and included hard data and open-ended material that was not covered in the General Schedule or other coding documents. Included in the Narrative Report were a description of patient, the reason for admission, his present illness, past medical history, past life history, and future outlook. Verbatim responses were recorded to get some of the flavor of the interview. The Narrative Reports on the patients were reviewed and each patient was given a score on the Accessibility Scale (see Table 19) based on his response. If a Narrative Report covered all or most of the questions and if the verbatim response were coherent and relevant, the patient was considered to be Completely Accessible. If a patient were able to respond to only a few of the questions or gave

Table 19

PATIENTS' ACCESSIBILITY

		N	%
Completely Accessible:			
Answers all questions relevantly, coherently, appropriately.[a]		137	26
Partially Accessible:			
Answers some questions appropriately, but cannot remember, falsifies, or responds inappropriately to others.		177	33
Inaccessible:		188	35
Grossly confused. Answers all or most questions inappropriately or cannot answer because of memory loss, delusion, etc.	135	25	
Language barrier or physical handicap	11	2	
Mute or comatose	22	4	
Refused all or most questions	20	4	
Unknown		32	6
Total		534	100

[a] Includes patients who refused or failed to respond appropriately in only one area.

some inappropriate responses, he was considered to be Partially
Accessible. Comatose or completely disoriented patients who were
unable to give an appropriate response to most or all of the questions were considered to be Inaccessible. A few patients who refused
the interview (4 per cent) or who were unable to respond because
of a language barrier or physical handicap (2 per cent) also were
considered Inaccessible.

DESCRIPTION OF INACCESSIBLES

Our analysis of the inaccessible patients was concerned with
their condition at baseline only. We wanted to find out whether
Inaccessibles were distinguished diagnostically from other patients,
what were the effects of age, sex, and socioeconomic status, how
much more dependent on others were the Inaccessibles for social
and physical support and what would be the probable outcome for
the older patient who was inaccessible when he was admitted to
the psychiatric ward. We found that there were some age and sex
differences that made it necessary to stratify the sample by age and
sex when we looked at other variables. Women were more often inaccessible than men at less than the .01 level of significance. Among
women, the older were significantly less able to respond at the .001
level; this did not hold true for the men, although there was a
slight but statistically insignificant trend toward the older men's
being more inaccessible.

Socioeconomic status. The present socioeconomic status of
male Inaccessibles was slightly better than that of male Accessibles:
56 per cent of the former ranked above the median compared to
45 per cent of the latter. The reverse was true for the younger
females. The present socioeconomic status of fifty-seven per cent of
the younger female Inaccessibles placed them above the median
compared with 64 per cent of the Accessibles. However, the ranking of the Partially Accessible younger women who were less well off
than the Inaccessibles clouded the findings, so that the slight relationship between present socioeconomic status and accessibility,
for the younger females, was not linear. In the older females there
was no relationship between accessibility and present socioeconomic
status.

Self-maintenance scales. The association between a poor

score on the Social Self-Maintenance Scale and a rating of Inaccessible was high for the men and for the younger women. Approximately nine-tenths of the inaccessible men and the younger inaccessible women were below the median on Social Self-Maintenance Scale while only one-fourth of the accessible men and younger accessible women fell below the median. Although the number of older accessible women was small, they were more likely to score below the median on the Social Self-Maintenance Scale than were either the younger women or the men. There was also a direct relationship between accessibility and the Physical Self-Maintenance Scale for all males and for both age groups of the females. The relation, however, was somewhat weaker than with Social Self-Maintenance Scale, with approximately one-fourth of the Inaccessibles in each group ranking above the median.

Psychiatric diagnosis. A diagnosis of chronic brain syndrome was predominant among male Inaccessibles (87 per cent, compared to 33 per cent of the male Accessibles), and among the younger female Inaccessibles (78 per cent had a chronic brain syndrome diagnosis, compared to only 24 per cent of the younger female Accessibles). The difference between the male Inaccessibles and the younger female Inaccessibles was attributed to the occurrence of superimposed acute brain syndromes; 51 per cent of the male Inaccessibles had both acute and chronic brain syndromes versus 28 per cent of the younger female Inaccessibles. In the older female Inaccessibles, chronic brain syndrome without acute brain syndrome was found only a little more frequently than with acute brain syndrome (51 per cent versus 42 per cent). In general, for patients with chronic brain syndromes, a superimposed acute brain syndrome was more frequently associated with inaccessibility among males and accessibility among females.

First follow-up location. The Accessibility Scale was a moderately good predictor of location status at the first follow-up. After one year 20 per cent of accessible males had died and 62 per cent were in the community. Sixty-four per cent of the inaccessible males had died, and 11 per cent were in the community. As only 15 per cent of the younger female patients died within the first year after admission, the emphasis for location status prediction shifts from death to psychiatric facility. Eight per cent of accessible younger females were in a psychiatric facility, and 87 per cent were in the community after one year. Fifty-five per cent of inaccessible younger females were in a psychiatric facility, and 17 per cent were in the community. The relation between location and the Accessibility Scale was not quite as strong for the older females. Fifty-eight per cent of the older accessible females were in the community and 16 per cent had died, while of the older Inaccessibles 16 per cent were in the community and 43 per cent had died.

SUMMARY

Women were more often inaccessible than men, and older women (seventy-five and over) were more often inaccessible than younger women (under seventy-five). Male Inaccessibles were somewhat more likely to be above the median on present socioeconomic status than were younger female Accessibles; older females showed no relationship between accessibility and present socioeconomic status. Male and female Inaccessibles were likely to be below the median on both the Social Self-Maintenance Scale and present socioeconomic status. Male Inaccessibles usually had diagnoses of chronic brain syndromes, mostly with a superimposed acute brain syndrome. Female Inaccessibles also had diagnoses of chronic brain syndromes, but the majority were without superimposed acute brain syndromes. After a period of one year, 64 per cent of the male Inaccessibles had died, 25 per cent were in a psychiatric facility, and 11 per cent were in the community. After the same period, 28 per cent of the female Inaccessibles had died, 55 per cent were in a psychiatric facility, and 17 per cent were in the community.

APPENDIX D

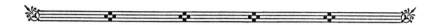

Other Statistical Tables

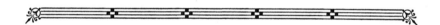

The following tables have not been included in the text for purposes of economy and brevity. Readers interested in procuring these mimeographed tables should address their requests to the Adult Development Research Program, 1415 Fourth Avenue, San Francisco, California, 94122.

CHAPTER 1: BACKGROUND CHARACTERISTICS OF THE PATIENTS

Samples Compared with the Elderly of San Francisco: Sex, Age, and Income

1E   Matched Subsamples from Hospital and Community Samples: Socioeconomic and Physical Characteristics

1F   Matched Subsamples from Hospital and Community Sample: Psychiatric, Self-Maintenance, and Social Characteristics

1G   Los Angeles and San Francisco Counties: Comparison of Elderly Population in General with Those State Hospitalized: Sex and Age

Chart

1A   Matched Subsamples from Hospital and Community Samples: Number of Months from Interview to Death

CHAPTER 2: POST-ADMISSION ASSESSMENT OF THE PATIENTS

2A   Precipitating Psychiatric Condition (ungrouped) by Sex and Age

2B   Per Cent Positive Responses to Fourteen Psychopathological Symptoms by Sex and Age

2C   Kent E-G-Y by Level of Orientation

2D   Per Cent Positive Responses to Sixteen Physical Complaints by Sex and Age

2E   Psychosocial Variables by Sex and Age

CHAPTER 4: COMPONENTS AND CORRELATES OF
PSYCHIATRIC STATUS

4A   Interrelationship of the Indicators of Psychiatric Status

4B   Degree of Psychiatric Impairment by the Indicators of Physical Status

4C   Number of Reported Psychopathological Symptoms by the Indicators of Physical Status

4D   Precipitating Psychiatric Condition by the Indicators of Physical Status

4E   Level of Orientation by the Indicators of Physical Status

4F   Degree of Psychiatric Impairment by Low Self-Maintenance

4G   Number of Reported Psychopathological Symptoms by Low Self-Maintenance

CHAPTER 6: RELATION BETWEEN PATIENTS' CONDITION
AT ADMISSION AND OUTCOME

APPENDIX E

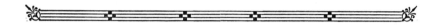

Selected Program
Publications

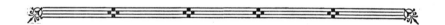

The reader is referred to the following selected publications based on this research program. They report on materials only briefly alluded to in this volume, including the intellectual functioning of the mentally ill aged.

BUEHLER, J. A. "Two Experiments in Psychiatric Interrater Reliability." *Journal of Health and Human Behavior*, 1966, 7, 192–202.

CAHAN, R. B., AND YEAGER, C. L. "Admission EEG as a Predictor of Mortality and Discharge for Aged State Hospitalized Patients." *Journal of Gerontology*, 1966, 21, 248–256.

CHRIST, A. "Attitudes Toward Death Among a Group of Acute Geriatric Psychiatric Patients." *Journal of Gerontology*, 1961, 16, 56–59.

CLARK, M., AND ANDERSON, B. G. *Culture and Aging: An Anthropological Study of Older Americans.* Springfield, Illinois: Charles C Thomas, 1967.

CROOK, G. H., AND KATZ, L. "Intellectual Functioning of Aged Patients and Nonpatients." In Tibbitts, C., and Donahue, W. (Eds.) *Social and Psychological Aspects of Aging.* New York: Columbia University Press, 1962.

EPSTEIN, L. J. "Institutional Planning." In Simon, A., and Epstein, L. J. (Eds.) *Aging in Modern Society,* Psychiatric Research Report No. 23. Washington, D.C.: American Psychiatric Association, 1968.

EPSTEIN, L. J., AND SIMON, A. "Alternatives to State Hospitalization for the Geriatric Mentally Ill." *American Journal of Psychiatry,* 1968, *124,* 955–961.

EPSTEIN, L. J., AND SIMON, A. "Prediction of Outcome in Geriatric Mental Illness." In Lowenthal, M. F., and Zilli, A. (Eds.) *Interdisciplinary Topics in Gerontology: Colloquium on Health and Aging of the Population,* Vol. 3. New York: S. Karger, 1969.

EPSTEIN, L. J., AND SIMON, A. "Social, Psychological and Physical Factors in Mental Health and Illness in Old Age." In *Proceedings of the 7th International Congress of Gerontology: Vienna, Austria, June 26–July 2, 1966,* Vol. 6. Vienna: Verlag der Wiener Medizinische Akademie, 1966.

FISHER, J., AND PIERCE, R. C. "Dimensions of Intellectual Functioning of the Aged." *Journal of Gerontology,* 1967, *22,* 166–173.

FISHER, J., AND PIERCE, R. C. "A Typology of Mental Disorder in the Aged." *Journal of Gerontology,* 1967, *22,* 478–484.

JAMBOR, H., "A Comparative Analysis of Employment Patterns of Older Psychiatric Male Patients and Men in the Community." In Tibbitts, C., and Donahue, W. (Eds.) *Social and Psychological Aspects of Aging.* New York: Columbia University Press, 1962.

KATZ, L., AND CROOK, G. H., "Use of the Kent E-G-Y with an Aged Population." *Journal of Gerontology,* 1962, *17,* 186–189.

LOWENTHAL, M. F. "Some Social Dimensions of Psychiatric Disorders in Old Age." In Williams, R. H., Tibbitts, C., and Donahue, W. (Eds.) *Processes of Aging: Social and Psychological Perspectives,* Vol. 2. New York: Atherton Press, 1963.

LOWENTHAL, M. F. *Lives in Distress: The Paths of the Elderly to the Psychiatric Ward.* New York: Basic Books, 1964.

LOWENTHAL, M. F. "Antecedents of Isolation and Mental Illness in Old Age." *Archives of General Psychiatry,* 1965, *12,* 245–254.

LOWENTHAL, M. F. "The Relationship Between Social Factors and Mental Health in the Aged." In Simon, A., and Epstein, L. J. (Eds.) *Aging in Modern Society.* Washington, D.C.: American Psychiatric Association, 1968.

LOWENTHAL, M. F., AND BERKMAN, P. L. "The Problem of Rating Psychiatric Disability in a Study of Normal and Abnormal Aging." *Journal of Health and Human Behavior,* 1964, *15,* 40–44.

LOWENTHAL, M. F., BERKMAN, P. L., AND Associates. *Aging and Mental Disorder in San Francisco: A Social Psychiatric Study.* San Francisco: Jossey-Bass, 1967.

LOWENTHAL, M. F., AND HAVEN, C. "Interaction and Adaptation: Intimacy as a Critical Variable." *American Sociological Review,* 1968, *33,* 23–30.

LOWENTHAL, M. F., AND SIMON, A. "Mental Crises and Institutionalization Among the Aged." *Journal of Social Issues,* in press.

LOWENTHAL, M. F., AND TRIER, M. "The Elderly Ex-Mental Patient." *International Journal of Social Psychiatry,* 1967, *13,* 101–104.

LOWENTHAL, M. F., AND ZILLI, A. (Eds.). *Interdisciplinary Topics and Gerontology: Colloquium on Health and Aging of the Population,* Vol. 3. New York: S. Karger, 1969.

MALAMUD, N. "A Comparative Study of the Neuropathologic Findings in Senile Psychoses and 'Normal' Senility." *Journal of the American Geriatrics Society,* 1965, *13,* 113–117.

SIMON, A. "An Approach to the Study of Geriatric Mental Illness." In *Proceedings of Seminars, 1959–61,* Duke University Council on Gerontology. Durham, North Carolina: Regional Center for the Study of Aging, 1962.

SIMON, A. "Mental Health of Community Resident vs. Hospitalized Aged." In Simon, A., and Epstein, L. J. (Eds.) *Aging in Modern Society,* Psychiatric Research Report No. 23. Washington, D.C.: American Psychiatric Association, 1968.

SIMON, A., AND CAHAN, R. B. "The Acute Brain Syndrome in Geriatric Patients." In Mendel, W. M., and Epstein, L. J. (Eds.) *Acute Psychotic Reaction,* Psychiatric Research Report No. 16. Washington, D.C.: American Psychiatric Association, 1963.

SIMON, A., AND EPSTEIN, L. J. "Organic Brain Syndrome in the Elderly." *Geriatrics,* 1967, *22,* 145–150.

SIMON, A., AND MALAMUD, N. "Comparison of Clinical and Neuropathological Findings in Geriatric Mental Illness." In *Psychi-*

atric Disorders in the Aged, Report on the Symposium held by the World Psychiatric Association at the Royal College of Physicians, London, England, September 28–30, 1965. Manchester, England: Geigy [1968].

SIMON, A., AND NEAL, M. W. "Patterns of Geriatric Mental Illness." In Williams, R. H., Tibbitts, C., and Donahue, W. (Eds.), *Processes of Aging: Social and Psychological Perspectives,* Vol. 1. New York: Atherton Press, 1963.

SIMON, A., AND TALLEY, J. E. "The Role of Physical Illness in Geriatric Mental Disorders." In *Psychiatric Disorders in the Aged,* Report on the Symposium held by the World Psychiatric Association at the Royal College of Physicians, London, England, September 28–30, 1965. Manchester, England: Geigy [1968].

SIMON, A., BERKMAN, P. L., AND EPSTEIN, L. J. "Psychiatric Screening of the Elderly." Paper presented at the 7th International Congress on Mental Health, London, England, August 12–17, 1968.

SPENCE, D. L., FEIGENBAUM, E. M., FITZGERALD, F., AND ROTH, J. "Medical Student Attitudes Toward the Geriatric Patient," *Journal of the American Geriatrics Society,* 1968, *16,* 976–983.

TRIER, T. R. "Characteristics of Mentally-Ill Aged: A Comparison of Patients with Psychogenic Disorders and Patients with Organic Brain Syndromes." *Journal of Gerontology,* 1966, *21,* 354–364.

TRIER, T. R. "A Study of Change Among Elderly Psychiatric Inpatients During Their First Year of Hospitalization." *Journal of Gerontology,* 1968, *23,* 354–362.

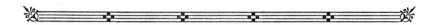

Bibliography

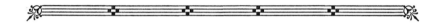

American Psychiatric Association. *Diagnostic and Statistical Manual of Mental Disorders*. Washington, D.C.: American Psychiatric Association, 1952.

American Psychiatric Association. *Diagnostic and Statistical Manual of Mental Disorders*. (2nd ed.) Washington, D.C.: American Psychiatric Association, 1968.

ARTH, M. J., WEST, J., BLAU, D., AND KETTELL, M. "Family Disinterest as a Factor in the Mental Hospitalization of the Aged." Paper presented at the 14th Annual Meeting of the Gerontological Society, Pittsburgh, Pennsylvania, November, 1961.

BLALOCK, H. *Social Statistics*. New York: McGraw-Hill, 1960.

BLAU, D. "The Role of Community Physicians in the Psychiatric Hospitalization of Aged Patients." Paper presented at the 14th Annual Meeting of the Gerontological Society, Pittsburgh, Pennsylvania, November, 1961.

BLAU, D. "Psychiatric Hospitalization of the Aged." *Geriatrics*, 1966, *21*, 204–210.

BLAU, D., ARTH, M. J., KETTELL, M., WEST, J., AND OPPENHEIM, D. J.

"Psychosocial Reasons for Geriatric Hospitalization." In Tibbitts, C., and Donahue, W. (Eds.) *Social and Psychological Aspects of Aging.* New York: Columbia University Press, 1962.

BLAU, Z. S. "Structural Constraints on Friendships in Old Age." *American Sociological Review,* 1961, *26,* 429–439.

BLENKNER, M. "Developmental Considerations and the Older Client." In Birren, J. E. (Ed.), *Relations of Development and Aging.* Springfield, Ill.: Charles C Thomas, 1964.

BLENKNER, M. "Environmental Change and the Aging Individual." In *Proceedings of 7th International Congress of Gerontology, Vienna, Austria, June 26–July 2, 1966,* Supplement, Vol. 8. Vienna: Verlag der Wiener Medizinischen Akademie, 1966.

BOTWINICK, J. *Cognitive Processes in Maturity and Old Age.* New York: Springer, 1967.

California, State of, Department of Mental Hygiene, Statistical Research Bureau. *Older Patients in California State Hospitals for General Psychiatry, 1959.* 1960a.

California, State of, Department of Mental Hygiene, Bureau of Private Institutions. *Private Institutions Licensed by the Department of Mental Hygiene for Fiscal Year July 1, 1959–June 30, 1960.* Sacramento, California: California State Printing Office, 1960b.

California, State of, Department of Mental Hygiene. *Statistical Report for the Year Ending June 30, 1960.* Sacramento, California, 1960c.

California, State of, Department of Mental Hygiene. Memorandum from Bureau of Biostatistics, August 9, 1968.

CLARK, M. "Positive or Negative Evaluations in the Self-Image of Mentally-Ill Aged." California Department of Mental Hygiene, No. 151, April 1963.

CLARK, M., AND ANDERSON, B. G. *Culture and Aging: An Anthropological Study of Older Americans.* Springfield, Illinois: Charles C Thomas, 1967.

CORSELLIS, J. A. N. *Mental Illness and the Ageing Brain,* Maudsley Monograph No. 9. London: Oxford University Press, 1962.

CROOK, G. H., AND KATZ, L. "The Intellectual Functioning of Aged Patients and Nonpatients." In Tibbitts, C., and Donahue, W. (Eds.) *Social and Psychological Aspects of Aging.* New York: Columbia University Press, 1962.

DOVENMUEHLE, R. H., NEWMAN, E. G., AND BUSSE, E. W. "Physical

Problems of Psychiatrically Hospitalized Elderly Persons." *Journal of the American Geriatrics Society,* 1960, *8,* 838–846.

EPSTEIN, L. J., AND SIMON, A. "Alternatives to State Hospitalization for the Geriatric Mentally Ill." *American Journal of Psychiatry,* 1968, *124,* 955–961.

EPSTEIN, L. J., AND SIMON, A. "Prediction of Outcome in Geriatric Mental Illness." In Lowenthal, M., and Zilli, A. (Eds.) *Interdisciplinary Topics in Gerontology: Colloquium on Health and Aging of the Population,* Vol. 3. New York: S. Karger, 1969.

FISHER, J., AND PIERCE, R. C. "Dimensions of Intellectual Functioning of the Aged." *Journal of Gerontology,* 1967a, *22,* 166–173.

FISHER, J., AND PIERCE, R. C. "A Typology of Mental Disorders in the Aged." *Journal of Gerontology,* 1967b, *22,* 478–484.

FREEMAN, H. E., AND SIMMONS, O. G. *The Mental Patient Comes Home.* New York: Wiley, 1963.

GELLERSTEDT, N. "Zur Kenntnis der Hirnveränderungen bei der normalen Altersinvolution." *Upsala Läk.-Fören. Förh.,* 1933, *38,* 192–408.

GIBSON, A. C. "Psychosis Occurring in the Senium." *Journal of Mental Science,* 1961, *107,* 921–925.

GOLDFARB, A. I. "Mental Health in the Institution." *The Gerontologist,* 1961, *1,* 178–184.

GOLDFARB, A. I. "Prevalence of Psychiatric Disorders in Metropolitan Old Age and Nursing Homes." *Journal of the American Geriatrics Society,* 1962, *10,* 77–84.

JASNAU, K. F. "Individualized Versus Mass Transfer of Non-Psychotic Geriatric Patients from Mental Hospitals to Nursing Homes, with Special Reference to the Death Rate." *Journal of the American Geriatrics Society,* 1967, *15,* 280–284.

KAHN, R. L., GOLDFARB, A. I., POLLACK, M., AND GERBER, I. E. "The Relationship of Mental and Physical Status in Institutionalized Aged Persons." *American Journal of Psychiatry,* 1960, *117,* 120–124.

KATZ, L., NEAL, M. W., AND SIMON, A. "Observations on Psychic Mechanisms in Organic Psychoses of the Aged." In Hoch, P. H., and Zubin, J. (Eds.) *Psychopathology of Aging.* New York: Grune and Stratton, 1961.

KATZ, L., AND CROOK, G. H. "Use of the Kent E-G-Y with an Aged Population." *Journal of Gerontology,* 1962, *17,* 186–189.

KAY, D. W. K., NORRIS, V., AND POST, F. "Prognosis in Psychiatric Disorders of the Elderly: An Attempt to Define Indicators of Early Death and Early Recovery." *Journal of Mental Science,* 1956, *102,* 129–140.

KAY, D. W. K., AND ROTH, M. "Environmental and Hereditary Factors in the Schizophrenias of Old Age ('Late Paraphrenia') and Their Bearing on the General Problem of Causation in Schizophrenia." *Journal of Mental Science,* 1961, *107,* 649–686.

KENT, G. H. "Kent E-G-Y Test." *Series of Emergency Scales.* Manual. New York: Psychological Corporation, 1946.

KNUPFER, G. *Characteristics of Abstainers: A Comparison of Drinkers and Non-Drinkers in a Large California City.* Berkeley, California: California Department of Public Health, Division of Alcoholic Rehabilitation (Report No. 3), November, 1961.

KNUPFER, G., AND ROOM, R. "Age, Sex, and Social Class As Factors in Amount of Drinking in a Metropolitan Community." *Social Problems,* 1964, *12,* 224–239.

KRAMER, M., TAUBE, C., AND STARR, S. "Patterns of Use of Psychiatric Facilities by the Aged: Current Status, Trends, and Implications." In Simon, A., and Epstein, L. J. (Eds.), *Aging in Modern Society,* Psychiatric Research Report No. 23. Washington, D.C.: American Psychiatric Association, 1968.

LIEBERMAN, M. A. "Depressive Affect and Vulnerability to Environmental Change in the Aged." In Jeffers, F. C. (Ed.) *Proceedings of Seminars, 1961–65.* Duke University Council on Gerontology. Durham, North Carolina: Regional Center for the Study of Aging, 1965.

LOCKE, B. Z., KRAMER, M., AND PASAMANICK, B. "Mental Diseases of the Senium at Mid-Century: First Admissions to Ohio State Public Mental Hospitals." *American Journal of Public Health,* 1960, *50,* 998–1012.

LOWENTHAL, M. F. *Lives in Distress: The Paths of the Elderly to the Psychiatric Ward.* New York: Basic Books, 1964a.

LOWENTHAL, M. F. "Social Isolation and Mental Illness in Old Age." *American Sociological Review,* 1964b, *29,* 54–70.

LOWENTHAL, M. F. "Antecedents of Isolation and Mental Illness in Old Age." *Archives of General Psychiatry,* 1965, *12,* 245–254.

LOWENTHAL, M. F. "Social Adjustment in the Aged." In *Proceedings of 7th International Congress of Gerontology, Vienna, Austria, June 26–July 2, 1966,* Supplement, Vol. 8. Vienna: Verlag der Wiener Medizinischen Akademie, 1966.

LOWENTHAL, M. F., AND BERKMAN, P. L. "The Problem of Rating Psychiatric Disability in a Study of Normal and Abnormal Aging." *Journal of Health and Human Behavior,* 1964, *15,* 40–44.

LOWENTHAL, M. F., BERKMAN, P. L., AND Associates. *Aging and Mental Disorder in San Francisco: A Social Psychiatric Study.* San Francisco: Jossey-Bass, 1967.

LOWENTHAL, M. F., AND TRIER, M. "The Elderly Ex-Mental Patient." *International Journal of Social Psychiatry,* 1967, *13,* 101–114.

LOWENTHAL, M. F., AND ZILLI, A. "Introduction." In Lowenthal, M. F., and Zilli, A. (Eds.) *Interdisciplinary Topics in Gerontology: Colloquium on Health and Aging of the Population,* Vol. 3. New York: S. Karger, 1969.

MCNEMAR, Q. *Psychological Statistics.* (2nd Ed.) New York: Wiley, 1955.

MALAMUD, N. "Mental Disorders of the Aged: Arteriosclerotic and Senile Psychoses." Supplement 168. *Public Health Reports,* 1942.

MALZBERG, B. "A Statistical Review of Mental Disorders in Later Life." In Kaplan, O. J. (Ed.) *Mental Disorders in Later Life.* (2nd Ed.) Stanford, California: Stanford University Press, 1956.

MILLER, D., AND LIEBERMAN, M. A. "The Relationship of Affect State and Adaptive Capacity to Reaction to Stress." *Journal of Gerontology,* 1965, *20,* 492–497.

NORRIS, V. *Mental Illness in London.* London: Chapman and Hall, 1959.

PIERCE, R. C. "Note on Testing Conditions." *Journal of Consulting Psychology,* 1963, *27,* 536–537.

POLLACK, E. S., LOCKE, B. Z., AND KRAMER, M. "Trends in Hospitalization and Patterns of Care of the Aged Mentally Ill." In Hoch, P. H., and Zubin, J. (Eds.) *Psychopathology of Aging.* New York: Grune and Stratton, 1961.

PUBLIC LAW 89–97, 89TH CONGRESS. H. R. 6675, July 30, 1965. *Social Security Amendments of 1965.*

RAHE, R. H., AND HOLMES, T. H. "Life Crisis and Disease Onset. II: Qualitative and Quantitative Definition of the Life Crisis and Its Association with Health Change." Unpublished paper, 1966a.

RAHE, R. H., AND HOLMES, T. H. "Life Crisis and Disease Onset. III: A Prospective Study in Life Crises and Health Changes." Unpublished paper, 1966b.

ROTH, M., TOMLINSON, B. E., AND BLESSED, G. "Correlation Between

Scores for Dementia and Counts of 'Senile Plaques' in Cerebral
Grey Matter of Elderly Subjects." *Nature*, 1966, *209*, 109–110.

ROTHSCHILD, D. "Pathologic Changes in Senile Psychoses and Their
Psychobiologic Significance." *American Journal of Psychiatry*,
1937, *93*, 757–788.

SEIDNER, F. J. *Health Insurance for the Aged.* Washington, D.C.: Public Affairs Institute, 1960.

SHELDON, H. D. "Changes in Family Composition and the Housing of
the Older Population in the United States." Paper presented
at the International Social Science Research Seminar in
Gerontology, Markaryd, Sweden, August, 1963.

SIEGEL, S. *Nonparametric Statistics for the Behavioral Sciences.* New
York: McGraw-Hill, 1956.

SIMON, A. "An Approach to the Study of Geriatric Mental Illness,"
Proceedings of Seminars, 1959–61, Conference on Gerontology,
November 19–21, 1959, Duke University Council on Gerontology (Durham, North Carolina: Regional Center for the Study
of Aging at Duke University, 1962), 174–192.

SIMON, A., BERKMAN, P. L., AND EPSTEIN, L. J. "Psychiatric Screening
of the Elderly." Paper presented at the 7th International Congress on Mental Health, London, England, August 12–17, 1968.

SIMON, A., EPSTEIN, L. J., AND REYNOLDS, L. "Alcoholism in the Geriatric Mentally Ill." *Geriatrics*, 1968, *23*, 125–131.

SIMON, A., AND MALAMUD, N. "Comparison of Clinical and Neuropathologic Findings in Geriatric Mental Illness." In *Psychiatric
Disorders in the Aged,* Report on the Symposium held by the
World Psychiatric Association at the Royal College of Physicians, London, England, September 28–30, 1965. London:
World Psychiatric Association [1968].

SPENCE, D. L., FEIGENBAUM, E. M., FITZGERALD, F., AND ROTH, J. "Medical Student Attitudes Toward the Geriatric Patient." *Journal
of the American Geriatrics Society*, 1968, *16*, 976–983.

SROLE, L. "Social Integration and Certain Corollaries." *American
Sociological Review*, 1956, *21*, 709–716.

THOMPSON, W. E., STREIB, G. F., AND KOSA, J. "The Effect of Retirement on Personal Adjustment: A Panel Analysis." *Journal of
Gerontology*, 1960, *15*, 165–169.

TRIER, T. R. "Characteristics of Mentally-Ill Aged: A Comparison of
Patients with Psychogenic Disorders and Patients with Organic
Brain Syndromes." *Journal of Gerontology*, 1966, *21*, 354–364.

TRIER, T. R. "A Study of Change Among Elderly Psychiatric Inpatients

During Their First Year of Hospitalization." *Journal of Geron-tology,* 1968, *23,* 354–362.

TRYON, R. C. *Identification of Social Areas by Cluster Analysis.* Berke-ley, California: University of California Press, 1955.

United States Bureau of the Census. *United States Census of Popula-tion, California, Detailed Characteristics,* Washington, D.C.: Government Printing Office, 1960.

United States Public Health Service. *Patterns of Retention, Release and Death of First Admissions to State Mental Hospitals.* (Monograph No. 58) Washington, D.C.: Government Printing Office, 1959.

WECHSLER, D. *WAIS Manual: Wechsler Adult Intelligence Scale.* New York: Psychological Corporation, 1955.

WHITTIER, J. R., AND KORENYI, C. "Selected Characteristics of Aged Patients: A Study of Mental Hospital Admissions." *Compre-hensive Psychiatry,* 1961, *2,* 113–120.

WILLIAMS, R. H. "Changing Status, Roles and Relationships." In Tib-bitts, C. (Ed.) *Handbook of Social Gerontology.* Chicago: University of Chicago Press, 1961.

Index

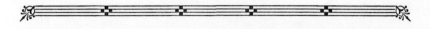